PRAISE FOR ALEXANDER KRISS'S *BORDERLINE*

"Thoroughly researched and beautifully written, *Borderline* will be of value to anyone interested in what is to this day one of the most challenging and complex psychiatric disorders."

—CHRISTOPHER CHRISTIAN, PhD, editor in chief,
Psychoanalytic Psychology

"*Borderline* is a gripping, humane, brilliantly prismatic inquiry into the peculiarities of the mind, at once a case study, an intellectual history, and a reckoning with the education of a therapist."

—ADAM EHRLICH SACHS, author of *Inherited Disorders:
Stories, Parables & Problems*

"*Borderline* is nothing short of a revelation. . . . [It] offers a compassionate and deeply insightful analysis of the ways that such patients have been dismissed, wronged, silenced, and deemed 'untreatable' by medical systems for many centuries—and, perhaps most importantly, it provides clear reasons why there is hope for such patients going forward."

—MARIN SARDY, author of *The Edge of Every Day:
Sketches of Schizophrenia*

"Insightfully and plausibly rendered . . . A revealing exploration of borderline personality disorder and the future of therapies addressing it."

—*KIRKUS REVIEWS*

"An enterprising and in-depth exploration of who decides what it means to be ill, how mental illness is framed in cultural narratives, and who gets shut out of those narratives. It's an ambitious reassessment of an understudied condition."

—*PUBLISHERS WEEKLY*

"A dialectical treat . . . Strikingly successful in underscoring the relevance of a contemporary psychoanalytic approach to psychotherapy but will be of interest to anyone who is curious about what happens in psychotherapy."

—ELLIOT JURIST, PhD, author of *Minding Emotions:
Cultivating Mentalization in Psychotherapy*

ALEXANDER KRISS, PhD

BORDERLINE

THE BIOGRAPHY OF A PERSONALITY DISORDER

BEACON PRESS
BOSTON

BEACON PRESS
Boston, Massachusetts
www.beacon.org

Beacon Press books
are published under the auspices of
the Unitarian Universalist Association of Congregations.

28 27 26 25   8 7 6 5 4 3 2 1

This book is printed on acid-free paper that meets the uncoated paper
ANSI/NISO specifications for permanence as revised in 1992.

Text design and composition by Kim Arney

The contents of this book are not intended to provide diagnoses or
advice on medical or mental health problems. The information provided
should not be used for diagnosing or treating a psychological or medical
problem, and those seeking personal advice for such a problem should
consult with a licensed physician or mental health professional.

*Library of Congress Cataloguing-in-Publication
Data is available for this title.*
ISBN: 978-0-8070-1659-6
E-book ISBN: 978-0-8070-0782-2
Audiobook: 978-0-8070-3527-6

For Zoe

When the voice that links the body to
the soul vanishes, there is no way to put
into words one's feelings or will. I am
reduced to pieces in no time at all.

—YOKO OGAWA, *The Memory Police*

CONTENTS

BORDERLINE

COLLECTIVE PSYCHOSIS

On April 26, 2022, clinical and forensic psychologist Shannon Curry took the stand at the Fairfax County Courthouse in Northern Virginia. She had been hired as an expert witness by the plaintiff, actor Johnny Depp, in a highly publicized defamation lawsuit he had brought against his ex-wife, actor Amber Heard. After the dissolution of their brief marriage, Heard had publicly accused Depp of physical and emotional abuse. Her statements, according to Depp, were untrue, the machinations of a vindictive ex with an unstable personality, and he contended that she had irreparably damaged his reputation and thus his future financial prospects.

Curry testified that, after having evaluated Heard for fourteen hours over the course of two days, she believed that the defendant met the criteria for borderline personality disorder, or BPD. The current edition of the American Psychiatric Association's *Diagnostic and Statistical Manual of Mental Disorders* (*DSM*) describes this disorder as "a pervasive pattern of instability of interpersonal relationships, self-image, and affects, and marked impulsivity that begins by early adulthood and is present in a variety of contexts."[1]

"Would you agree that a disproportionate degree of women are tagged with a diagnosis of borderline personality disorder?" Heard's counsel asked Curry under cross-examination.[2]

"No, that's not quite right," Curry replied.

"Seventy-five percent?"

"The way you phrased it is not quite right."

"Tell me, tell me what's right."

"Okay, so there are more women who have been diagnosed with bipolar disorder [*sic*] than men; it's more prevalent in women," Curry said.

"And trauma can cause borderline personality disorder, can't it?"

"No."

"Never?"

"Right now, we know that there are people who have borderline personality disorder who have sustained childhood trauma," Curry said. "There are also people who have borderline personality disorder who have had no childhood trauma. So, like most personality disorders and, really, like most mental health issues in general, there seems to be both a biological component—in this case, with borderline personality disorder, the research tends to support a genetic component and possibly a neurological component, and then there is also possibly an environmental component triggering those genetic markers."

Through Curry's testimony, Depp's lawyers hoped to portray Heard as innately irrational, hysterical—as a person who sought to defame her ex-husband out of a predisposition to act crazy, rather than as a participant in a toxic dynamic for which Depp might also be held legally responsible. The jury's acceptance of this narrative was tangibly expressed a couple of months later when it determined that Heard owed Depp $15 million in compensatory and punitive damages, while Depp—whom Heard had countersued—owed Heard only $2 million in compensatory damages.

Almost everything Curry said in her testimony was incorrect. Yet, while Heard's counsel pushed back some, no one was prepared to fully defy Curry's presumed authority regarding psychological illness, as the version of reality she presented was in full accordance with mainstream views on BPD.

Never mind the questionable legitimacy of giving a personality disorder diagnosis to someone after having known her for only two days. Never mind Curry's dismissal of the rate of women versus men diagnosed with BPD—well documented in the *DSM* and elsewhere. Never mind that Curry had mistakenly used the term "bipolar disorder" when she meant BPD, betraying a common confusion among mental health providers that often leads to those diagnoses being conflated and misapplied. Never mind Curry's flagrant misrepresentation of scientific evidence: contemporary research suggests that, at most, 40 percent of the variance in borderline cases can be attributed to biological factors, leaving 60 percent to the environment.[3]

Perhaps most of all, never mind Curry's unequivocal denial of the relationship between BPD and trauma. Given the media frenzy that had erupted around *Depp v. Heard*, even a conservative estimate would suggest that tens of millions of people heard that particular exchange, spoken by a doctor under oath.

"And trauma can cause borderline personality disorder, can't it?"
"No."

When *Depp v. Heard* began, I had already been working on this book, an attempt to reconsider the chronically misunderstood and much maligned borderline, for a couple of years. This book emerged on a scale more intimate than that very public trial's, with a comment made by a patient in my private psychotherapy practice, whom I refer to throughout this book as Ana. (All of the patients I describe are based on real people, with identifying information removed or changed to protect their privacy.)

"Everything I've read about what it means to be borderline describes people at their most extreme," Ana said. Why, she asked, were people with BPD never depicted in a state of change, of growth? Innumerable books and articles on other conditions found in the *DSM*—such as depression, anxiety, and explicitly trauma-based disorders—highlighted the process of healing and recovery. Did BPD's exclusion from this company mean the condition really could not be treated? This has not been Ana's or my experience of the disorder, even though—or perhaps because—my approach to working with her fell outside the present mainstream of psychology.

I am a psychoanalytic psychologist. This means some things you might expect—I have a couch in my office and see some patients three or four times a week—and others you might not. I don't oblige anyone to lie down during sessions, and in fact discourage many patients from doing so—especially those who I think would benefit from staying grounded in the reality of the session, in the back-and-forth of words and facial expressions. I don't tell patients what to call me. Most settle on "Alex," though some stick with "Dr. Kriss" even after knowing me for months or years. Often this speaks to how a patient thinks of the power dynamic in our relationship: Are we equals on a first-name basis or am I a "doctor"? Are they my client or my patient? I tend to use the terms interchangeably, though I prefer the latter for its association to someone in pain seeking help; the former has always struck me as too sterile and businesslike to describe psychotherapy as I understand it.

For me, the psychoanalytic approach is less about what I do as how I think. It means I believe in unconscious motivation—that there are parts of ourselves we cannot directly access that nevertheless influence our thoughts, feelings, and behaviors. It means I'm reluctant to take simple explanations of the human condition—even when delivered by figures of authority like Shannon Curry—at face value. Perhaps most of all, it has come to mean for me the belief in a fundamental truth: that, at our core, we are all psychotic.

By "psychotic" I do not mean inherently delusional; I mean that we all possess an internal world unbound by time, social rules, or logic. A place of raw emotion with no names or borders—where emotion is the logic. We were all born screaming into this world, without words or understanding. We have all known the abject terror of hunger and the enveloping satiety of feeding at the breast or bottle. We don't remember these first experiences of being human—before we have language to articulate the things that happen to us, we create very few memories at all—but they have been with us longer than anything else we might identify as ourselves.

Psychosis only becomes a diagnosis when it appears at times or in places we deem unacceptable. Children are frequently psychotic—that is, immersed in their internal world—but in ways we expect and therefore see as appropriate: they talk to imaginary friends; they get confused about whether things on TV are real or make-believe; they become so overwhelmed with emotion that they throw themselves to the ground, kicking and screaming. Adults continue to make contact with their psychotic core from time to time. Dreams are the most ubiquitous example: a nightly experience that is still poorly understood by science; a space we briefly inhabit that is no space at all; a derivation of us that we cannot consciously influence, where events make the purest kind of sense while we are asleep and then, upon waking, seem like nonsense.

There is no firm line between sanity and insanity. We all live on a shared continuum; our place on it varies by the extent that we learn to impose order on the psychotic chaos into which we are all born. Some people, through a complex interaction of genes and environment, fall toward one end of this continuum, struggling to form the mental structures that allow them to reliably distinguish dreams from reality. For these people, their waking logic retains the boundlessness of the psychotic core. We tend to refer to these people as ill and give them labels like "schizophrenia." Others manage to create the necessary structures to distinguish inside from outside. They create these structures so well, in fact, that they come to believe there is only one real world, the external one where we have friends and jobs, schedules and budgets. We tend to refer to these people as normal.

Many of us exist on this "normal" end of the continuum. We are extremely sane, which is to say extremely rigid: in a desperate bid to lay claim to our normalcy, we deny the psychosis that is part of us. We refuse to accept that some parts of the human experience will always be out of our conscious control. Above all, we reduce the continuum to a binary—the ill and the well, the crazy and the sane—and in so doing lose track of the multitudes living somewhere in the middle. We don't tend to know what to call these lost souls, though they are all around us. Indeed, some of us are them.

In the past four thousand years, they have gone by many names. The ancient Greeks called them hysterical; medieval priests called them sorcerers and witches. In 1890, alienist* Irving Rosse, in an almost frightened tone, called them a "vast army . . . with minds trembling in the balance between reason and madness," and for whom contemporary medicine was almost entirely unhelpful.[4] Today, we say these people have BPD.

BPD is what happens when a person is denied a history. Usually this occurs because of chronic abuse or neglect beginning early in life: the instinct to survive, to predict catastrophe at the hands of an unpredictable authority figure, takes up all the space that might otherwise be devoted to learning who you are. Eventually BPD binds you to the present, so that every feeling seems permanent, every thought inescapable. Time cannot heal wounds because time does not exist; emotions can only be resolved through action.

The borderline experience is typically depicted from an outsider's perspective, portraying wild, promiscuous people—usually women— who abuse substances, threaten suicide, and fly into rages. This cliché is accurate for some, not for others. For many, the borderline experience is unremarkable from the outside—they look like us, they *are* us, with jobs and friends, if not always a schedule and budget. Their suffering can only be known from the inside, where life is an endless sprint: toward anyone who promises to validate, to define, to love; away from the terrifying emptiness that always seems poised to well up from within and dissolve one's sense of self into nothing.

---

*A nineteenth-century term for physicians specializing in the treatment of mental disorder, later replaced by the more familiar term "psychiatrist."

This is a book about what it actually means to live on the borderline: what it has meant from antiquity to the present day, what it means for patients who are diagnosed, and what it means for doctors like me who assign diagnoses. It's about what we can learn from accepting that the borderline experience exists, to some degree, in all of us.

To look at BPD is to confront who we are and who we have been. It is the displacement onto individuals of our collective fears about madness and losing control. It is the systematic blaming of women, ignoring of children, and obscuring of chronic abuse that people in power have long relied on to maintain their status. It is the pain inflicted by denying history, and it is the hope that can come from picking up the severed threads of the past and attempting to tie them back together. It is the individual manifestation of society's search for meaning and identity.

Perhaps this search is in vain. Perhaps there is no way out of the cycle in which we have found ourselves for thousands of years, hurting those who most need help and absolving those most responsible for causing pain. Perhaps we are destined to make the same mistakes over and over. But, then again, perhaps not.

PREHISTORY

The First Session

T he morning began with a dead sparrow on my doorstep, its breast ripped open. It was a sight that some people might have interpreted as an omen for the coming day. I was of no such persuasion. An existentialist by nature and a clinical psychologist by training, I was a skeptic twice over. While, as Sigmund Freud said, inside our heads there's no coincidence—only unconscious connections we've yet to unearth—the outside world is full of coincidence.[1] Stuff happens every day, all the time, indifferent to the designs of people who, for thousands of years, have tried to assign intent to random events. Despite my training as a psychoanalytic psychologist, I did not take everything Freud said as gospel—my relationship with him and the tradition he birthed was complicated—but I took as inviolate his assertion that all experience was filtered through the mind. I looked on the sparrow with pity and no small measure of disgust, but the story of how it arrived at my door felt as unimportant as it was unknowable. Donning dishwashing gloves, I placed the bird into a trash bag, tossed the bag into the bin on the curb, and continued on my way to work.

The first half of my day proceeded as usual, seeing a series of patients in my small private office in downtown Manhattan. When Ana, a new patient whom I'd not yet met, arrived for her first session, I had little idea what to expect. She had emailed me the week before with the subject line, "Call me ASAP," and the body text, "I'm looking for a therapist that will guide me, not tell me what to do. Just left an abusive relationship . . . need help sorting this out." Despite her directive to call—or maybe because of it—I responded by email, offering Ana a mid-afternoon Thursday slot that I'd had trouble filling. I suppose a part of me didn't want to meet her at all, because I did have *some* idea what to expect. Even in our brief correspondence I'd felt an intensity, a static discharge coming off the computer screen.

When Ana arrived for her appointment, I showed her into the office and invited her to sit down. She was in her late twenties with a round, ashen face framed by ringlets of black hair—a combination, I would later learn, of Spanish-Mexican ancestry on her father's side and Anglo-American ancestry on her mother's. Ana dressed in black: my immediate thought was of a veiled woman in mourning, though her face was uncovered. When she began to tell me her story, her words indicated a fierce intelligence and poetic sensibility, but not all of what she said made conventional sense. Ana revealed that she had been raped two weeks earlier by her boyfriend, Tom, and that she was in the process of having, in her words, a total nervous breakdown. She said she did not want to go to the police but did want to hold Tom accountable. It became clear that the situation was blurrier than indicated in her email, in which she'd written that the relationship was over. On my notepad I tallied each time she used the phrase *I don't want to leave*. By the end of our session I'd made nearly a dozen hashmarks.

I asked Ana how she had been doing since the rape, and she began with a report of expectable symptoms: poor sleep, racing thoughts, panic. She listed these off in a way that suggested I was not the first therapist she had spoken with since the assault. But her anxious energy, combined with my relative silence, soon steered her into territory less practiced, less controlled.

Ana paused and her eyes darted about the room. She said she wondered if the rape hadn't been *owed* to her, and she leaned in as she said this, which caused me to lean back. When I asked what she meant, she described a dream she'd had in which a spirit had spoken to her of a "horrible dowry," a lineage of pain and sexual abuse passed from her grandmother to her mother to her.

"I know it was only a dream," she said, "but it was actually a big reason I decided to give therapy a try. I saw on your website that you're interested in psychoanalysis, which I know has a lot to do with interpreting dreams."

I felt disoriented. When she'd first spoken of the dream she seemed to sincerely believe that it was a kind of prophecy—but now she seemed just as sincere in her effort to convince me that it was no more than a by-product of her unconscious mind. I wasn't sure who she was trying to convince.

I told her to go on, because I didn't know what else to tell her, and the dizzying narrative intensified, like a whirlpool carrying us closer to its center. Ana explained that she had been a diligent vegan for the past several years but that last week she'd decided she *needed* to eat a hamburger. She said she believed ingesting animal flesh would help to replace what Tom had scooped out of her. When she said "scooped out," my skin erupted in goose pimples. I reflexively checked my arms to confirm they were sleeved, as though I ever wore anything but long sleeves to work. Ana described the act of eating the fast-food burger she had bought, its juices dripping down her chin.

"I felt like a wolf," she said.

I remembered the dead sparrow. Had I really found it on my doorstep that morning, or was it part of a dream I'd had during the night? Or was I conjuring the image now, for the first time, and confusing it for a memory?

Ana said she realized everything she was saying sounded "insane," that of course she knew a hamburger was just a hamburger.

Again, her about-face led me to doubt whether what I had just experienced was real. Ana said the ritual of eating meat was a symbolic gesture and not a literal reclaiming of her physical body. She did not use the word "transubstantiation," but I thought of it—I, a secular Jew who believed that the mind created God and not the other way around. I thought of the Athenian dramatist Euripides, whom I'd studied as a playwriting major in college. Two and a half millennia ago, his play *The Bacchae* depicted a group of women driven mad by the god Dionysus. They were said to have torn a cow to pieces with their bare hands.[2]

I did not speak these thoughts aloud. Nor did I share the image that flashed before my mind's eye: of Ana, feral and transformed, carrying a dead sparrow in her mouth, depositing it at my doorstep. *Like a wolf,* she had said.

I struggle to recall when I first heard the term "borderline personality." Most likely as an undergrad at New York University, during the Abnormal Psychology class I took as part of my psychology minor. (Though the term "abnormal" has been excised from most graduate psychology programs, it is still used in many undergraduate departments to refer to mental illness. Change, as we will see, is nonlinear and slow.) I also hold a vague memory from around that same time of my friend and classmate Beth telling me she had been diagnosed with BPD. But it's possible I've invented that part of the story to fit my later understanding of what she might have been going through. Who we are now has a way of inserting itself into the stories of who we used to be.

My relationship with Beth was never sexual, yet it had an undeniably romantic quality. I felt drawn to her by a pull so strong that it defied my so-called better sense. She was funny in a way that now I might call mean: you wouldn't want to be the target of her vitriol, but I found pleasure in watching it burn someone else. She drank to excess most nights, while I tended toward violent hangovers after just a few beers; often, I would look out for her at the bar or dorm party until she goaded me to drink past my limit, and then she would take care of me. A week might pass when we'd barely speak and I would never know why. We had almost no friends in common.

Sometimes Beth would ping me on AOL Instant Messenger in the middle of the night. Her messages often began innocuously—"Hey"— but could quickly turn into an ultimatum: I needed to respond to her or she would kill herself. I would get upset and tell her not to put me in that position, which still qualified as a response, and the next morning she would act as though nothing remarkable had transpired between us. In truth, a part of me liked feeling needed by Beth in the way that she needed me: immediately, absolutely, and then hardly at all.

At the start of my junior year I left New York to study abroad for four months, and it felt as though the spell were broken. I didn't yet know of the history connecting witchcraft and witch hunts to borderline conditions—even so, I made contact with that history, feeling myself free of Beth's thrall and, when I thought about it, frightened to return to her. I received an email from her a few weeks before we would both be in New York again, stating that she had all but fallen apart without me and that she eagerly awaited our reunion.

I replied to say that things had changed for me since I went away; that I valued our friendship but could no longer be what she wanted me to be, which seemed to be everything. A few hours later she responded tersely, suggesting I was being melodramatic—and, even more, that I had mistaken our whole relationship as more serious than it ever was.

"I just thought it would be nice to grab a coffee, but have it your way," she concluded.

The next time I saw my therapist—who I'd been working with since I was fifteen—I told him I felt confused and embarrassed. Had I completely misjudged the situation?

"You drew her attention to something she wasn't ready to look at," he said. "She's allowed to save face."

I barely saw Beth after that, and we lost touch completely after college. I've always remembered my therapist's take on our falling out, though. What feels like an attack is often the other person's attempt at self-protection.

Is that where my history with BPD began? It doesn't explain the magnetism I felt toward Beth. I must have seen in her something familiar, a kind of person I'd known all my life. Someone I wanted, or wanted to be wanted by, or felt compelled to save. But humans created diagnosis to separate the familiar from the alien, the normal from the abnormal. It's clear to see that Beth was unwell when I knew her. But then, I suppose that makes it clear that I was unwell too.

A year out of college I began my graduate studies in psychology at The New School, also in New York City. To some it seemed like a sharp pivot from playwriting, but to me it felt like a natural progression: my interest in narratives and human relationships merging with the transformative experience of my own therapy. The first two years of graduate school were all courses in "general psychology," a euphemism denoting the study of the normal: development (how do normal children grow), cognitive neuroscience (how do normal brains work), social psychology (how do normal people engage with one another), perception (how do normal people see, smell, hear, and touch). In my third year I began my study of the clinical—that is, the abnormal, the ill—and also started working as a therapist in the field. My first placement was on an adult inpatient psychiatric unit at Beth Israel Medical Center in Manhattan, which was also the first place I encountered someone who I knew to be officially diagnosed with BPD.

My supervisor at Beth Israel was a psychologist named Helena—she was young, knowledgeable, and extremely serious. She advised us against speaking about our work or patients anywhere outside of the unit. She said we were now representatives of a sacred but misunderstood profession and you never knew who might overhear you in an elevator or at a coffee shop or walking down the street. So the next time you felt the urge to giggle with a classmate in a public place about some "crazy" patient, remember that if a stranger overheard you, and then that stranger avoided treatment in the future for fear of being mocked behind his back, and then one day, God forbid, he killed himself—well, that would be on you.

Helena's view struck me as severe, but I was in awe of her confidence in a world I was only beginning to know, so I tried to live by her creed as much as possible. Though most of my contact with her was in the privacy of her office—debriefing the events of the group therapy sessions I had led earlier that week—sometimes we would walk the halls of the eighteen-bed unit together and, in hushed tones, she would offer insights on patients as we passed them by.

"Look at him," she said once as we approached a decrepit man using a walker, with rotten teeth and yellowed eyes. "That's what opioid addiction looks like. He's twenty-five years old."

As with everything else, Helena took this part of her job seriously, introducing a new recruit to the realities of acute mental illness. It was an awesome responsibility, teaching someone to navigate the mania, psychosis, and catatonia from which the general public was shielded, conditions relegated to faceless, fluorescent halls like the one she and I walked together. During one group session I asked a middle-aged Black man, diagnosed with paranoid schizophrenia and recently admitted to the unit, to introduce himself. He stared at me for a moment and said, "You already know me. I'm the guy out there digging for cans and food. The crazy homeless guy. The trash man. Maybe you've never really *seen* me, but you know me!"

I devoured whatever morsels of insight Helena gave me to make sense of the madness in which I was suddenly ensconced. Not only the madness of mental illness, but of the institution itself. Watching nurses remove their take-out containers from a medical fridge just before a health inspection, only to return them straight after. Listening to one of the unit's psychiatrists pass judgment on a patient's "unhealthy lifestyle," only to see him outside the main entrance an hour later chain-smoking like his cigarettes were about to be confiscated. Seeing an agitated patient strapped to a bed by his arms and legs. These were not peculiarities of that hospital, I would later learn, but a larger inverted reality that takes shape anytime one group is tasked with judging another group's right to be free.

Helena was right to take her job so seriously: her students looked to her to shepherd them through this terrain, and I quickly came to take her word as gospel. Erasmus said that in the land of the blind, the one-eyed person reigns, which I don't mean as a dig at Helena—I respected her then and I still respect her now. But it's hard to work on a psych ward with more than one eye open.

One day, walking the unit, Helena pointed out a white woman in her forties lounging on the floor with her back against the wall, legs splayed out into the middle of the hall. As a nurse passed by, stepping carefully over this woman's outstretched limbs, I could hear the woman ask him for an extra blanket. "Not for me," she clarified, pointing to an open door across the hall. "My roommate is cold."

Helena stopped us out of earshot and turned to me. "That woman does not belong here," she said.

"What do you mean?" I asked.

"She came into the ER last night, saying she was suicidal. Does she look depressed to you?"

"I don't know. I guess she looks relaxed."

"She's borderline. She knew just what to say to get admitted, and now she's going to try to control the unit, to manipulate staff and patients. It's going to take us a few days to get her out of here, so be mindful."

"Should I not invite her to groups?"

Helena paused. "I can't tell you not to invite a patient to group. But let's say you don't need to ask twice."

The patient, who went by Jo, did not need to be asked twice—she was first into the group room with me later that day. I did an exercise with the patients that I had been experimenting with all year, taken from my undergraduate days studying creative writing:

a group member would write one sentence of a story on a piece of paper, then pass the paper to the next member, who would write the next sentence to continue the story. At the end we would read the whole thing and talk about it. Though patients' writing skills and ability to follow a linear narrative could vary widely, in the best cases we ended up with a beautiful collaboration that evoked myriad thoughts and feelings, leaving the group with the sense that they had accomplished something meaningful together.

That day, I began the story with the line, "I woke up to the sound of the phone ringing." I passed the paper to Ricardo, a man grappling with depression and drug abuse who had been on the unit many times before. He wrote, "It was my dealer and I told him to go away." After reading this contribution aloud, he passed the page along to Nina, a woman with delusions and a moderate intellectual disability who had been on the unit much longer than most, as her social worker struggled to find a safe place to discharge her. She read her line aloud: "I called friends and family to say what happened, they said we'll be right there."

Jo received the paper next. She tapped the pencil on the laminate table for a moment, thinking, then wrote her sentence. She picked up the page with a flourish and read out, "Unfortunately, they all died in a car crash on the way over." She slid the paper to the next patient.

In an instant, the group fell apart. Nina began to sob. Ricardo shook his head and attempted to console her. The other patients complained that Jo had made it impossible for them to advance the story. They all looked to me. It was all I could do to mask the fact that I was as angry as they were.

"Let's give Jo a chance to explain what she meant," I said.

Jo feigned ignorance at the reactions around her. "I thought this was a creative writing assignment," she said. "I was using my imagination."

"This is group therapy," I replied, "and you were being provocative."

There was a pregnant pause. Jo stood up suddenly from her chair, scraping it along the linoleum floor and making us all flinch. "Whatever," she said, and headed for the door. Usually the idea in these groups was to encourage patients to stay, even if there was conflict, so that the issues at hand might be explored and worked through. I made no attempt to stop Jo. As she passed my chair on the way out, she looked at me and said, "You're terrible at this."

At the time, the whole episode felt like proof of Helena's earlier assessment: Jo did not belong; she wanted to mess with people; she was not really suffering. By the time I was next on the unit a few days later, Jo had been discharged, and I can't say that I thought of her again—not until I dug up the piece of paper with that brief story on it from the bottom of my files. Because now, more than a decade later, I *wanted* to remember—I could see how myopic I had been. I hadn't wanted to understand Jo. I'd wanted her to leave me and my nice little group alone.

But what kind of person *wants* to be admitted to a psychiatric inpatient unit? She may not have been truly suicidal, but something had brought her there. What was she running from? And even if she had been consciously trying to stir the pot . . . why? Who wants to be hated by a room full of people? And how had I ever convinced myself that someone who wrote about their friends and family dying in a car crash was not suffering?

I see now that in those early days, Helena's perspective compelled me not for its accuracy but its simplicity. *This is what opioid addiction looks like. This is what mania looks like. And this, this one here, this is nothing at all.* Jo was not a patient, she was a problem. We couldn't help her, so we needn't feel bad when, inevitably, we didn't.

There were others. The middle-aged woman I saw in a community clinic, who generated such confusion and disagreement among the staff that a special conference was held to discuss the case. The student I worked with for a few months at a college counseling center, who said that when we made eye contact she felt as though her insides were being torn out. The young man I saw for two years who constantly tried to please me yet often left me feeling disgusted.

Despite having completed years of what I consider excellent clinical training, by the time I met Ana—in my private office, no longer protected by the hierarchies of mental health institutions—I still didn't entirely know what I or anyone else meant by "borderline." Yet even in that first session, the word entered my mind, as though primed. Where had BPD come from? Surely it hadn't emerged out of whole cloth in the 1970s, when the term "borderline personality" first appeared in professional writings. I had never heard a consensus around even the most basic questions about it. Was BPD treatable and, if so, how? Did it represent an experience on a continuum with other mental disorders, or something unto itself? Was Ana in danger? Was I?

As I neared the end of our first session, feeling exhausted and confused, Ana and I turned to logistics.

"My boyfriend will be paying for this," she said, reaching into her handbag.

"You mean Tom?" I asked. Not even *ex*-boyfriend, now. As though progressing through the session had sent us backward in time.

"Yes," she said, hackles rising. "He owes me that much, at least. Don't you agree?"

"I'm more concerned about depending on someone who abused you for treatment. Sometimes people think they're entitled to know about the things they pay for. Could you afford this without his help?"

Ana handed me the debit card she had been fumbling to extract from her purse.

"I'm telling you my rapist is going to pay your fees," she said, shaking her head. "You must think I'm fucking crazy."

I took the card from her and looked at it. A wolf gazed out at me from beneath the familiar logo of a major bank. It struck me that I'd gotten it all backward.

"You want to be like this wolf," I said. "The lone hunter. The frightening creature of the night. But you're not. You're a woman who has experienced a terrible trauma. It must feel," I said, thinking of the dead sparrow, "as if you've already died of an open wound."

This, it bears mentioning, was quite a bit more phantasmagoric than I typically aim for in a patient's first session, especially as I'm essentially ushering them out the door. The words slipped out. I was unaccustomed to words slipping out. I was the kind of therapist who some considered too withholding, not too loose. But there had been a connection and, consciously or not, I had seized it: a sense that an experience I'd had before ever meeting Ana was somehow, inexplicably, a part of her experience as well. For a moment the world felt small and intentional, and it terrified me.

Ana stared at me, nodding. She mouthed the word "yes," but no sound came out. Her eyes were wet with tears. I swore I could see myself reflected in those shimmering mirrors.

2

SPLITS, HYSTERIA, AND THE INVENTION OF PSYCHOTHERAPY

Fifth Century BCE–1885 CE

On the wall of my childhood bedroom hung an autostereogram, better known as a Magic Eye poster. The trick to the poster's illusion, which took more hours to master than I'd care to admit, was to simultaneously relax and focus on the two-dimensional image—to not look at the thing it seemed you were supposed to look at—so that a hidden, three-dimensional image (in this case, a rocket ship) emerged. Tracing the history of what we now call BPD recalls that struggle against intuition and reflex. It is confronting the absence of history, or the history of absence; it is finding the latent dimensionality in flat narratives. We humans aren't good at nuance; the space between categories makes us anxious, so we tell ourselves there is no space, that the space is an illusion, that what looks like space is actually just another category.

Reducing a continuum of experience to a binary is a common psychological defense that twentieth-century psychoanalysts called "splitting."[1] Splitting allows for no complexity, no shades of gray—something or someone is either all good or all bad. We split when it feels that good and bad must be kept apart—more specifically, to prevent the bad from infecting the good, like a drop of ink falling into a glass of water. In infancy, everybody splits; we lack the experiential or neurological maturity to do otherwise. A newborn cannot think as an adult can, cannot say to herself, "My mother loves me and feeds me when I'm hungry, but sometimes she's busy so I have to wait a few minutes before feeding can begin." All the baby knows is that sometimes she is hungry and sometimes she is sated. When sated, her love for the figure cradling her is boundless and uncomplicated; when hungry, she is filled with a desolation with which no parent can reason. Only as she grows up will she come to appreciate that the comforting mother she has loved and the absent mother she has hated are one and the same, complicated yet real.

Psychoanalytic therapists typically consider splitting as experienced by individuals, especially as a way for those with BPD to organize their experiences, a remnant of infancy held fast through the disruptions of abuse or neglect. But splitting is not simply a defense of the diagnosed or the very young. In the adult world, splitting is a way to justify mistreatment. If the target of abuse can be cast as wholly bad—not a person, but a whore, a witch, a lunatic—the abuser is absolved of guilt, even praised as right and just. These splits arise at a cultural level in order to promote simple stories that maintain the status quo over complex ones that challenge it. Because these splits are sanctioned by those in charge and accepted by large groups, they are not regarded as pathological. History itself cannot escape this compulsion; it is written by the victors, and thus the history of BPD is, perhaps above all else, the history of medical authority—of who decides what it means to be ill.

The first major compendium of illness is credited to the ancient Greek physician Hippocrates, who towers over the history of medicine despite lacking a known biography. Most likely, the body of work now known as the Hippocratic corpus (from which modern doctors'

"Hippocratic oath" is still derived) was penned by multiple authors over a protracted period of time, roughly from the late fifth to early fourth centuries BCE.[2] Like a game of telephone, the Hippocratics' knowledge of illness was passed on, cherry-picked, mistranslated, and otherwise transformed over centuries, from Roman physicians like Pliny the Elder and Galen of Pergamon to Arab and Jewish scholars in the Middle East through the Dark Ages, until returning home to Europe, recognizable yet changed, at the dawn of the so-called Enlightenment. Given these exchanges of knowledge across time and geographical space, the very notion of "the West"—with regard to the history of medicine or anything else—is worthy of our skepticism. I will nevertheless at times invoke "the West" as a shorthand for the perspectives that would come to dominate European and North American culture and, in more recent decades, exert a global influence—a viewpoint often defined by maleness and, eventually, whiteness. But I do not mean to suggest that the splitting of West and East is more than a narrative convenience. Even when consciously trying to avoid it, the pull of the split endures.

The Hippocratics were empiricists: they made meticulous observations of illness and the efficacy of treatment. A neglect of anatomy, however, limited their understanding of disease. In modern times, a patient presenting to a doctor with sharp pain in his lower right abdomen might be diagnosed with appendicitis, thanks to the doctor's understanding of how a malfunction in a specific part of the body—that is, the appendix—produces that sensation. The Hippocratics, by contrast, would have classified the same condition only by its observable symptom, *pónos*, meaning "pain."[3]

There was one notable exception. The Hippocratics posited that a great many symptoms reported by women—from epileptic-like seizures to stomach pain to the feeling of being choked—resulted from her uterus wandering about her body. Though many scholars would later state that the Hippocratics had invented a distinct diagnosis for ill or otherwise unstable women known as "hysteria," in fact their ancient corpus simply described a range of maladies using variations on the root word *hystera*, for "womb."[4] The con-solidation of female illness under that single name, as we will see, would come later. Nevertheless, this anatomical focus was unusual for the Hippocratics and a betrayal of their empirical philosophy: we know they never observed a womb moving about someone's body because we know wombs don't actually do that. Yet this theory helped to explain any vexing symptom an ancient Greek woman might present to an unfailingly male physician, as he could attribute her various experiences to her womb having roamed to various places. More importantly, it sowed a seed that would forever shape how we think about illness, especially mental illness: if a woman had a problem that a doctor didn't understand, it was assumed to owe to her *being* a woman.

The concept of a feminine disease did not occur to the Hippo-cratics in a vacuum. Depictions of women as unpredictable and bifurcated, often exemplified by the intermingling of sexuality and violence, were found throughout ancient Greek culture and in the Roman tradition that followed. Euripides wrote in his plays of the Bacchae tearing up cattle with their bare hands in a fit of religious ecstasy, and of Medea murdering her own children after being jilted by her lover. Homer sang of the Sirens, whose sole purpose in life was to lure men to their shore with heavenly voices, only to rend their flesh with beastly claws. Ovid wrote of Medusa, a lovely demigod who turned monstrous after being raped by the sea god Neptune, and whose gaze thereafter could turn mortal men to stone.[5]

Perhaps this dual vision of femininity represented the Hippo-cratics' observation of hysterical symptoms transmuted into myth. Or, perhaps the myths reflected a cultural expectation that women conform to one of two identities—being either subservient to men or frighteningly out of control, an expectation so pervasive that it came to shape a disorder.

———

In our modern era of information, and with the framework of so-cial justice, we see society's splits abstractly and often look upon them with judgment. Yes, the world is unfairly painted in black and white, but not by us. People with BPD do not have the luxury of this distance. They rely on the splitting of their experiences to survive and, in that reliance, sometimes draw uncomfortable attention to our collusion in the age-old practice of flattening the world into two dimensions.

When the public learned in 2017 that migrant children were being separated from their parents at the US-Mexico border and sent to detention facilities, Blake, a patient of mine with BPD, ob-served how aghast his peers were at the news. Then he summed up his position in two words.

"Fuck kids."

My jaw dropped. If Blake noticed, he continued as though I wasn't in the room.

"Everyone's saying we need to take better care of them. Why? They're being fed, they have a place to sleep. Kids don't know anything."

Psychotherapy is two people working together in a refinery. The patient passes raw material to the therapist, who must smelt it down to something usable. A part of me wanted to say to Blake, "I wonder how you'd like to be forced into a cage." But this would be handing the emotional ore straight back to him, unprocessed, rage for rage. At the same time, swallowing Blake's stance wholesale would also run counter to the goal of refinement. I could feel the anger radiating between us; to just say "I understand how you feel" would be more avoidant than empathic. Besides, I *didn't* understand.

"Don't you think," I asked slowly, "that these children are frightened?"

"So what if they are? This is my point. If an adult is scared, they can act on it. They might go out and do damage, hurt people. That's who we need to be worrying about. Kids are just kids. They need, need, need, but can't do anything. They don't matter."

I studied Blake's face. His guard was up. This organization of the world made sense to him and he was prepared to defend it. Children were undeserving; only adults had thoughts and feelings worthy of our consideration.

"But Blake . . ." I continued to screen each word as it left my mouth, for fear of lashing out at Blake before either of us really knew what we were talking about. "Eventually these kids will grow up."

He stared at me for a moment. His face softened. He looked embarrassed.

"I guess so," he said.

I sensed a relaxation in Blake's defenses, which emboldened me. "What they're being subjected to now will change how they see themselves and the world. Those changes might take them down paths they wouldn't have otherwise traveled. As adults they will be who they are, in part, because they lived through these experiences."

"Is that true, though? Do kids even remember the stuff that happens to them?"

This was a valid question. For Blake, I knew, memories of childhood felt imprecise, marked by the cataclysmic event of his father abandoning the family at age six, followed by Blake's mother traveling aimlessly around the country for years, children in tow, in search of emotional and financial stability.

"Maybe memory is more than what we consciously recall," I said. "Maybe you've come to this conclusion about children because of how you were treated as a child."

For Blake, the idea that a thread connected his past and present was novel. His father's abandonment had cut it, shocking and debilitating his mother, leaving six-year-old Blake to make sense of the loss. And because six-year-olds have a limited capacity for critical thinking, he faced the split: either Blake's father was bad for leaving, or Blake was bad and deserved to be left.

Children, when forced to make this choice, invariably pick the latter. They still depend on others for safety and sustenance, and so it is more adaptive to see the world as reliable and the self as corrupt.

Once grown, Blake started to regard all children as unlovable in an unconscious attempt to justify his father's actions and purge himself of a sense of rottenness. The splitting of child and adult kept a vision of the world intact—a distorted vision in which hurting children was sensible and carried no consequence—and held at bay the thought Blake had been trying not to think for twenty years: that abandonment by a parent forever alters a child's life, yet his father did it anyway.

Blake's position of "Fuck kids" first struck me as outrageous. But as our conversation took on shades of gray, it occurred to me it was, in a sense, mainstream—the imprisonment of children by the federal government being a painfully obvious testament to that fact. Blake saw his friends' moral outrage as hypocritical: they talked a good game but didn't act on their convictions beyond sharply worded Instagram posts. Though appalled by current events, I had been similarly inactive. I hadn't attended any related protests, donated money, or even written my congressman. We all belong to the same society, one that regards children as more disposable than adults, but Blake's friends and I had found ways to see ourselves as separate from that view, in order to allow ourselves to live and work without falling into despair. Blake's madness, then, was not so much his holding of contemptible opinions but his inability to compartmentalize them, reflect on them, or bury them into the recesses of his mind like the rest of us.

The borderline has lived a chameleon-like existence, blending into the nebulous space between whatever split dominated the mainstream culture of a given era. The Hippocratics split according to anatomy, in a time and place where the social and the physical were flip sides of the same coin—*gyne*, the Greek word for woman, is also the word for wife.[6] Bodily illness resulting from a woman's failure to conform to social norms therefore posed no contradiction. Neither was it considered overstepping for a Hippocratic physician to treat his female patient's illness by recommending that she marry and have sex with a man. Though this was not the only proposed treatment for hysterical problems, its impact across time and space cannot be overestimated. Here the idea was born that illness in women owes to their refusal to submit to the authority of men.

A shift away from splitting according to anatomy began in the second century CE, when the physician Galen of Pergamon took up the task of merging medical knowledge with metaphysical questions of the soul—launching, in essence, the field of mental health. Galen was born to a wealthy family in 129 CE in Pergamon, a site in modern-day Turkey that was a cultural epicenter of the Greco-Roman world. There he was exposed from an early age not only to Greek intellectual and religious thought, but also to Jewish theology and the scriptures of a nascent religious cult calling itself Christianity. Over the course of a storied career that included extended stints at the side of the emperor, Galen synthesized body and soul into a comprehensive theory of medicine, drawing heavily from the Hippocratics for his understanding of the former and from the ancient Greek philosopher Plato for the latter.[7]

Advances in anatomy and physiology led Galen to reject a wandering womb as the de facto explanation for female illness, though he upheld the essence of that hypothesis by continuing to link a wide swath of symptoms in women to their sex and sexuality. Galen viewed the failure to regularly engage in the "release" of sexual intercourse, rather than a nomadic organ, as the cause of female illness. In these cases Galen advocated for many of the same treatments found in the Hippocratic corpus, including the prescription of sex and marriage.[8] While there is limited evidence that he healed women with greater success than the Hippocratics, it is abundantly clear that Galen's theory of hysterical phenomena—that a woman's dysregulated internal "passion" led to bizarre and, at times, serious illness—informed his theory of "metaphysical disorder," or what we now call mental illness.

In his 180 CE treatise, *The Diagnosis and Cure of the Soul's Passions*, Galen outlined a new split to distinguish the sick from the

healthy—not between male and female anatomy, but between passion and reason. He defined passion as "an irrational power within
us which refuses to obey" and declared it the source of behavioral
dysfunction.[9] He went on to propose the following: if inexplicable
or unacceptable behavior results from excessive passion, and if
passion is an irrational force that has not been properly tamed by
reason, then perhaps conversing with a reasonable person would
help the afflicted to master his passions and improve his behavior.
Two people talk, one is relieved of suffering: here was the Western
world's first theory of psychotherapy.

Galen's work contained some ideas that read as shockingly modern, describing methods of managing anger and delaying impulsive
action wholly recognizable to a present-day psychotherapist. In one
recounted episode, Galen was approached by a friend from Crete
who was shirtless and with whip in hand, begging to be flogged
for a shameful act of violence he had committed earlier in Galen's
presence. Instead of gratifying this request for absolution through
physical pain, Galen spoke at length to his friend, lecturing him on
how to "train the irascible element within." The anecdote ended with
Galen winking slyly to the reader: "This is the way, obviously, that
I flogged him."[10] The talking cure was not without its discomfort,
Galen acknowledged, but it was through reasoned words, not bodily
punishment, that the pain of the soul could be soothed. He went on
to report that over the course of the next year his friend "became a
much better man," adding that even if the change had been slight it
would have been worth the effort.

Yet Galen was also bound by the social values of his day and
the hierarchies of male supremacy and slave ownership. Galen's
Cretan friend had savagely beaten a slave—which is why he faced
no punishment beyond his own guilt—and Galen also owned slaves.
True, he admonished his friend for his behavior, proudly referring to
a self-imposed injunction, passed down from Galen's father, "never
to strike any slave . . . with my hand." But he then quickly appended
this tenet, lest a modern reader confuse him for a social progressive,

by clarifying that anyone who abuses their slaves with fists in the heat of anger "could have waited a little while . . . and used a rod or whip to inflict as many blows as they wished . . . to accomplish the act with reflection."[11]

With respect to women, Galen espoused the mainstream perspective of their inferiority to men. Passion existed in men and women alike, but women—being of softer flesh and weaker nature—were more prone to both physical and metaphysical illness. Galen saw the ideal therapist as male and preferably advanced in age—to ensure that time and wisdom had freed him from passion's thrall—and the talking cure was presumed to be useful only for grown, free men seeking to improve themselves. When it came to matters of the soul, women were a lost cause. "Untamed horses," Galen wrote, "are useless."[12]

Ironically, the few surviving accounts of Galen putting his theory into practice occurred with women and slaves.[13] In one case, Galen uncovered that a woman's insomnia and physical restlessness were rooted in her being in love with an unavailable man. In another, he discerned that a slave's emaciation came not from physical illness but anxiety over having lost some of his master's money, and Galen proceeded to broker a truce of sorts between the two. His theory prioritized self-improvement of the ruling class, but in practice the oppressed apparently needed the help.

The origins of Galen's sexism are not difficult to fathom. Beyond its cultural normalcy in the Roman Empire, the work of his intellectual father, Plato, was rife with misogyny. In *Timaeus*, Plato proffered an origin story of humankind in which the first race consisted solely of men, and those who were too weak or corrupt to sustain that civilization came back in the second generation as women.[14] But Plato's work is also marked by contradiction. His mentor, Socrates, seemed to hold a more egalitarian view of the sexes, and Plato wrestled with advancing those ideas versus spreading his own bitterness, which some modern scholars have suggested stemmed from his being a gay man in a culture that prized male bisexuality.[15] History's game of telephone is as much a matter of selective attention as anything else: Galen absorbed Plato's misogynistic views uncritically while ignoring the contradictions and complications, including Plato's defense of male homosexual pederasty, of which Galen was no doubt aware.

What guided Galen's selective attention, or anyone's for that matter? We forgive much villainy by saying that an individual was only acting according to the values of their time. As an explanation for how human beings develop a sense of themselves and their values, however, doing so is as dismissive as calling someone with BPD "crazy."

In his treatise on the soul's passions Galen reflected on his childhood memories, one of the only known instances in which he did so among his voluminous writings. He drew a sharp contrast between growing up with his father—"the least irascible, the most just, the most devoted, the kindest"—and witnessing his mother's eruptions of anger and violence, including her biting her handmaid and spewing vitriol at the family.[16] From these experiences Galen arrived at an unambiguous conclusion. "When I compared my father's noble deeds with the disgraceful passions of my mother," he wrote, "I decided to embrace and love his deeds and to flee and hate her passions."[17]

Galen's mother counted among the untold victims of the split that had been codified centuries earlier by the Hippocratics. Galen, in turn, split himself. "Fuck kids," Blake told me, and two thousand years earlier Galen said, "Fuck feelings." His narrative formed: a weak mother swayed by passion and an unimpeachable father guided by reason. It was the understandable attempt of a frightened boy trying to make sense of the world around him. That this narrative persisted into Galen's adulthood, however, had profound consequences. By the time he was old enough to read Plato, Galen saw a version of himself in the text—and the parts he didn't recognize, he ignored.

Galen would have benefited greatly from his own talking cure, or a modified version of it not so firmly "of his time." Without a means of confronting the split, his immature worldview informed writings that would expand the pathologizing of women started by the Hippocratics and Plato, steering Western thought toward the idealization of logic, which Galen cast as masculine. He debased and feminized emotion—which he so desperately wanted to believe did not belong to him—confining it within the impulses of an unknowable mother.

The invention of psychotherapy is thus inseparable from one man's experience of early psychological trauma. Galen's work birthed a new split that empowered men and vilified women, that regarded men as being at their best when devoid of feeling, and women at their worst when resistant to male authority. The talking cure also introduced a question into the annals of human history, one that has since eclipsed the circumstances of Galen's personal life or the society in which he lived—a question with which we still wrestle: Can a relationship change who we are?

The Hippocratics and Galen gained authority through the accumulation of esoteric knowledge: few had access to the education and privileged social status that facilitated their rise in the nascent field of medicine. By the sixth century in Europe, the Catholic Church would gain this authority through fear. This was when the bubonic plague claimed an estimated one hundred million lives, an unfathomable loss inflicted by an invisible killer, in an era long predating knowledge of the microbe. In their terror, people shifted allegiances en masse from the Roman emperor's government, which offered little protection, to the Church, which, if not a cure, at least gave an explanation: humanity was being punished.

The plague catalyzed the next major shift in medical authority in the West: clergy became the de facto practitioners, guided by a new split. The ancient world's male-versus-female split, which had morphed to reason versus passion in Galen's time, now metastasized into the ultimate binary—good versus evil. Illness implied wickedness, and treatment meant accepting God's judgment: Catholic monks cared for the sick almost exclusively through prayer and bloodletting, both of them means of purging sin from the body.[18] Though women occupied a second-tier status in the Catholic Church, as they had in antiquity, for an extended period the Church did not treat them differently from men when it came to disease or unusual behavior. All sinned and bled equally, more or less. Any notions of "hysteria" disappeared.

Starting in the mid-fifteenth century, however, the status quo flipped on its head once again. Weary of the Church's iron grip on their finances and social order, European nations began to declare independence from the papal regime. By 1517, an emboldened German priest named Martin Luther publicly had accused the pope of exploitation and launched a so-called reformation of the Christian faith. To reestablish control, the Church needed a new plague—that is, something to serve as a scapegoat for society's ills and a reason to trust the pope's authority—or at least to fear defying it. Inspiration came from an unlikely source: an obscure, unfinished thirteenth-century text, previously decried as heretical, which claimed that demons walked freely among us by colluding with witches.

This text, the *Summa Theologica*, written by the Italian priest Thomas Aquinas, synthesized the ideas of the fifth-century theologian Augustine of Hippo—who contended that all humans were born wicked following the "original sin" of Adam and Eve—with the works of ancient Greek philosopher Aristotle, a student of Plato whose misogyny was even less inhibited than his mentor's.

Aquinas, a child of Sicilian aristocracy, had spent his youth as an outcast among seven athletic, military-bound brothers; by multiple accounts he was socially awkward and practically mute, referred to by classmates as "the dumb ox."[19] At age nineteen, he tried to flee his family castle to join the Dominican Order, an evangelical Catholic sect, only to have his mother physically confine him to his room in the hopes that Thomas would have a change of heart. A deep resentment grew instead—one that, like Galen's rejection of his mother's passion, would come to have profound cultural ramifications, even after Aquinas finally left Sicily to live as a Dominican friar for the rest of his life. How often, it would seem, that the course of human history has been set by men struggling to find peace with how their mothers treated them.

Women were a mistake, Aquinas wrote in the *Summa Theologica*, in an astonishing rebuke of God's design: "Nothing misbegotten or defective should have been in the first production of things. There-fore woman should not have been made at that first production."[20] Original sin, he asserted, was not an Adam and Eve problem—Eve, the temptress, had led Adam to sin and bore sole responsibility for the fall of humankind. Aristotle, whom Aquinas referred to simply as "the Philosopher," had argued that a woman's inherent inferiority made her subservience to man part of the natural, not merely social, order, and Aquinas carried this argument into the realm of Christian morality.[21] The ease with which a woman's soul could be corrupted by evil was more than a theological abstraction—it was, to Aquinas, an ongoing threat to public health and safety.

"When a soul is vehemently moved to wickedness," he wrote, "as occurs mostly in little old women . . . the countenance becomes venomous and hurtful, especially to children, who have a tender and most impressionable body. It is also possible that . . . spiteful demons cooperate in this, as the witches may have some compact with them."[22] This was the statement that fifteenth-century Catholic authorities would seize upon in their attempt to reestablish control over the European continent, and it would serve as the foundation for rewriting borderline phenomena for the next several hundred years. Evil was feminine, and madness in women was evidence of neither physical nor metaphysical illness, but of demonic possession.

This attitude was codified in a document called *Malleus Malefi-carum*, usually translated as "Hammer of Witches," published by two Dominican monks in 1486. The treatise argued that the seduction of women by the Devil was a pressing social problem and that the pope had the authority to put on trial anyone suspected of being a witch. Unsurprisingly, to modern eyes the document is rife with contradiction. Displays of excess emotion, sexuality, or physical fits—all historically associated with hysterical conditions—were grounds for suspecting witchcraft, but at the same time, a woman not showing adequate emotional upset during her trial was also considered verification of her being possessed.[23] Exorcism, first depicted in the Gospel of Mark as an act of healing conducted by Jesus Christ, was recast as the practice of banishing demons from the world by any means necessary—including executing its host body.

So began a three-hundred-year crusade against women. One record from 1586 reported a visit by inquisitors to a cluster of German villages; by the time they departed, all but two women had been tried, convicted, and murdered.[24] Men, too, were persecuted if they displayed hysterical symptoms or showed sympathy toward accused women. Identifying the ill and isolating them from the well—through public shaming, torture, or execution—overtook any priority the Church had ever placed on relieving people of suffering.

In truth, naming a disease had always been a greater sign of power than the ability to cure it. The Hippocratics had not always been able to heal the sick, but they'd had a name for every sickness. Galen's spotty track record of treating women did not prevent him from being viewed as an authority on the subject. When it came to inexplicable behavior, whether hysterical or heretical, effective treatment did not bestow authority. What mattered was giving the behavior a name.

As the medical field advanced through seventeenth- and eighteenth-century Europe, nosology—the science of classifying disease—became a religion in its own right among physicians: every condition under God's azure sky, every blister and boil, every disturbance of the spleen and infection of the liver, would be named. Even as effective treatments lagged behind, medicine's increasingly superior ability to name the suffering of human life came to challenge the Church's dominion over the continent's cultural split. Rather than good and evil, the line between sickness and health returned from antiquity to a place of prominence, while incorporating new ideas about anatomy, physiology, and heredity.

One of the greatest contributors to this movement was the seventeenth-century physician Thomas Sydenham. Textbooks now often refer to him as the "English Hippocrates," a moniker earned in large part through his tireless efforts to catalogue his patients' many ailments. One of these ailments would capture medical imagination for the next two centuries, with a name rooted in the ancient corpus beginning to resurface after a thousand years of darkness: hysteria.

It is worth noting that much of Sydenham's influence on hysteria and medicine in general came about posthumously.[25] During his lifetime, he practiced successfully but with only modest renown under a provisional license in the Westminster neighborhood of London. His writings were met with mixed reception. Sydenham had a reputation, valued by some and derided by others, for being more devoted to his patients than to winning the recognition of his peers; for experimenting with novel treatments to reduce suffering; and for speaking plainly to patients about the limits of medical knowledge. This should not surprise us, though perhaps its rarity in our story thus far should: the most thoughtful depiction yet of the borderline experience—an experience documented since the start of human history—would come from a doctor who cared about the people he treated.

Two observations by Sydenham cemented hysteria's position in the Enlightenment era and beyond as a mystery worthy of the medical field's sustained attention. First, he said that hysteria was exceedingly common—"no chronic disease occurs so frequently as this," he wrote.[26] Second, Sydenham saw hysteria's chameleon-like nature not as an impediment to its definition, but rather as its defining characteristic. He downplayed the emphasis others had placed on dramatic symptoms, like choking and epileptic fits—signs of a wandering womb to the Hippocratics, of excessive passion to Galen, and of demonic possession to Catholic monks. These were not the hallmarks of the condition, Sydenham said; what made hysteria unique was that its symptoms, whatever they were, broke the rules that physicians took as inviolate. A patient who presented as blind should not spontaneously recover her sight days later, for instance, yet Sydenham observed this phenomenon and countless others like it in his practice every day. *Hysteria disobeyed.* It was an illness that didn't behave like an illness should.

As physicians of the seventeenth century wrestled the 'borderline out of the pope's hands, they found themselves in need of their own theory of hysteria's etiology—that is, of where it came from. Sydenham and several of his contemporaries rejected the Hippocratic notion of a wandering womb, but the final abandonment of this two-millennia-old theory raised a question that few were interested in answering; If its cause was not found in female anatomy, was hysteria still a female disease?

As ever, Sydenham needed only to look to his patients for the answer—though it was an answer that would not hold the medical profession's attention like his other insights had. It would, rather, be lost again for centuries; for many it remains lost. Sydenham noted that while women presented certain symptoms of hysteria, like convulsions, more often than men, there were still plenty of men—especially those who led a "sedentary or studious life, and [grew] pale over their books and papers"—showing up with problems that made no medical sense.[27] They, too, complained of pains, emotional fits, or sudden onsets of sexual or aggressive behavior, none of which quite fit into other disease categories or responded to standard treatments. The issue, it seemed, was not that hysteria preferred women over men, but that physicians preferred to call it something different depending on the gender of the patient. Men tended to be labeled as hypochondriacs—another new and poorly defined term of the era—while women were overwhelmingly called hysterics. Beneath the labels, Sydenham wrote, these men and women differed like "one egg as to another."[28]

But unsexing hysteria was no easy task. If naming a thing was a sign of authority, *explaining* it carried responsibility. By the eighteenth century, hysteria's acceptance as a legitimate and common diagnosis meant that explaining its etiology was akin to taking a stance on the role of women in society, and on how female disobedience should be understood and treated.

Franz Mesmer, a German physician working in Vienna and France in the years leading up to the French Revolution of 1789, learned the price of trying to use medical authority to challenge the broader social order. Mesmer pioneered the use of hypnotism to treat hysteria based on his theory of "animal magnetism," which contended that a physical, invisible substance connected all matter in the cosmos, and that imbalances in this substance were responsible for the hysterical and hypochondriacal illnesses that other doctors couldn't explain. To correct these imbalances, Mesmer would induce a state of "waking sleep" on groups as large as twenty at a time—composed of men and women alike—and then use his hands or various instruments to "move" the alleged substance through the body without making physical contact, not dissimilar to the twentieth-century Japanese practice of reiki, which also claims a physiological basis.

Mesmerism was, from the vantage point of the present, a pseudoscience destined to collapse under its own weight. But in those tumultuous years in France, it was also an affront to systemic oppression. The idea that the cause of hysteria was a substance that was universally present—transcending gender, class, even humanity itself—drew consternation from the highest seats of power. In 1784, King Louis XVI commissioned an investigation into Mesmer, which concluded that Mesmer's theories of an ethereal substance could not be verified; even more, it denigrated his hypnotic treatment as trickery and manipulation. Mesmer was driven into exile, professionally disgraced until his death in 1815.[29]

For the first half of the nineteenth century, few were willing to stick their necks out to explain hysteria as Mesmer had, lest they too find the figurative guillotine awaiting them. The medical movement had, in the interim, cemented into an establishment, far-reaching and founded on the meticulous classification of disease advanced by Sydenham, now canonized as the second coming of Hippocrates. The Devil was definitively banished from the doctor's office, and in its place came a new split, more recognizable to our modern eyes than good and evil, though no less arbitrary: the split between sanity and insanity.

Individuals could be designated as insane due to a broad range of symptoms and behaviors, from hallucinations to hypersexuality, all of which butted against the strictures of polite society and, importantly, refused to yield to a physician's treatment. The insane were freed from the torture and humiliations of the Church only to be shuttled to the asylums of Western medicine: part prison, part experimental laboratory, part tourist attraction. And with this segregation came the beginnings of specialization in medicine: so-called alienists ruled over the asylums, while other physicians tended to the hearts, lungs, and gall bladders of those living free.

The one condition that could not fit neatly into this new split was, of course, hysteria. Who held title and deed over the illness that was not an illness? Who *wanted* it?

Everyone and no one—the paradox continued. On one hand, hysteria patients were lucrative: they had frequent, ever-shifting symptoms and continued to seek help even when treatments failed; the patient's reliance on medical authority and a willingness to pay for it seemed almost to be a feature of the disease. On the other hand, hysteria patients were infuriating: there was always a new problem; they never felt satisfied; they blamed their doctors when their condition failed to improve.

Physicians dealt with this tension in different ways. Some rejected the money, calling hysterical patients frauds and turning them away from their practices. Others treated hysterics for as long as they could bear, until a borderline was crossed, so to speak, and then they called in the alienists, who would take the patient away; hysteria rebranded as lunacy. Institutionalized life in nineteenth-century Europe—even after the so-called moral reforms of legendary French physician Philippe Pinel—remained rife with indignities: though no longer beaten or chained as in the earlier days of bedlam, patients faced overcrowding, poor living conditions, and a dearth of treatments. Above all, they faced a slim likelihood of returning to their former lives. When a physician, driven past the brink of frustration with a hysterical patient, referred her to be committed, he did so knowing full well his professional opinion held as much power as any judge—with the stroke of a pen he could indefinitely remove the offending woman from society.

Still other doctors channeled their rage at hysterical patients through the act of healing itself. One London doctor, W. Tyler Smith, in 1848 gleefully reported about his program of "injections of ice water into the rectum, introduction of ice into the vagina, and leeching of the labia and cervix."[30] He noted with something approaching wonder how quickly the leeches sated themselves.

Smith tortured his patients, at least in part, as punishment for their apparent refusal to get better. The alternative would have been to entertain the intolerable notion that he lacked the knowledge or skill to treat them. This may be less a relic of the past than we'd like to believe. Many professionals working today behave in accordance to Smith's driving principle: they don't believe you can do anything for someone with BPD, and in their disbelief they perpetuate the abuses of the past. I have met with patients—in the twenty-first century—who, before seeing me, had been told by another doctor that they were "incurable," or were destined to hurt other people; that they would die alone, or spend the rest of their lives drifting in and out of mental institutions, as disposable as a plastic bag.

Research shows that people with BPD are frequently misdiagnosed, especially with bipolar disorder.[31] This error can trigger the prescription of strong psychotropic drugs like lithium that confer little to no benefit to borderline symptoms while risking serious side effects. Bipolar disorder, properly diagnosed, often responds well to these treatments; clinicians must contend with the urge to force what their patient presents into the shape of something they know how to handle.

A patient of mine once met with a psychiatrist—who, as opposed to a clinical psychologist like me, is trained and licensed to prescribe medications—to talk about a possible prescription for the anxiety she would experience when flying. After reviewing her initial paperwork, in which she had disclosed the BPD diagnosis I had given her, he declared, "You can't be borderline. You're too likable." My patient, dumbstruck, said that she believed the diagnosis was correct, but that she was in a good place and had been helped by therapy. "That's also not possible," the doctor said, and nothing more.

Where, meanwhile, were the "sedentary and studious" men who Sydenham had found indistinguishable from hysterical women? The weird men holed up in their rooms, like Thomas Aquinas bathing himself in the works of Aristotle? In the Dark Ages they had been a rare breed and had been treated as such—any man who had time for books while there was still fighting and farming to be done was surely a sorcerer. But as academic and government bureaucracy exploded in the subsequent Renaissance and Enlightenment eras, barreling toward industrialization, men were in greater and greater numbers called away from the fields of agriculture and war to be ushered into a new social class that had scarce resemblance to traditional masculine roles. These men, like so many women since the days of antiquity, were expected to obey: to do their administrative jobs, collect their wages, fulfill their limited function within the great machine of a now-secular society. They lived well but controlled little, and so learned the importance of keeping a mild manner, an obsequiousness, of not biting the hand that fed. They were civilized; they were broken. "Untamed horses are useless," Galen had said.

These men, too, bothered their doctors to no end. They were given all manner of pills and tinctures: bogus treatments, though perhaps less nakedly sadistic than those bestowed on their female counterparts, designed not so much to heal as to shut them up. Men who presented with inexplicable physical symptoms were called hypochondriacs, as in the days of Sydenham, while those exhibiting the more behavioral side of hysteria—aggressive outbursts, like Galen had observed in his mother; pivots into sexual depravity; rapid shifts from despondency to giddiness—were given a new name: "moral insanity."

English physician James Cowles Prichard coined the term in 1835 to capture those individuals who seemed at once to be intellectually reasonable and emotionally mad. Untethered from questions of female behavior or anatomy, Prichard wrote one of the first recognizable ancestors of the modern BPD diagnosis: the morally insane were often educated models of civility, he stated, and yet struck by "morbid perversions of the feelings" so strong that they bled into patients' behavior, defying social norms and risking confinement to an asylum.[32] On paper, these individuals led respectable lives. In reality, they fought, fornicated, and spent recklessly; they provoked great distress in close friends when their affirmations of love turned suddenly to declarations of hatred. Often, these patients were not considered ill at all until a sudden violent act—Prichard cited a famous Pinel case in which a wealthy young man, feeling slighted, threw a woman down a well—landed them either in bedlam or prison.

Prichard did not specify moral insanity as a male disorder, yet almost all the case studies his treatise inspired were of male patients. No one in particular noticed the resemblance to contemporaneous case studies of female hysteria. And, as with hysteria, there was no cure for moral insanity. Those who tended toward violence eventually wound up imprisoned or committed; the more restrained cases would, as American alienist Irving Rosse wrote in 1890, "ultimately become the prey of quacks and charlatans."[33]

By the turn of the twentieth century, interest in Prichard's diagnosis was fading. Contemporary medical writings reveal an implicit sexism: many physicians argued that the symptoms of moral insanity simply weren't medical at all, an argument no one made when identical symptoms were labeled as hysteria in women. Experts seemed to agree that men were predisposed to sanity—their struggles were moral and metaphysical, issues that René Descartes had argued belonged firmly outside the realm of science in his influential seventeenth-century treatise *Meditations on First Philosophy*. So, as far as medical authority was concerned, morally insane men could go to a prison or be taken in by "quacks and charlatans." Or, if it so pleased them and they could afford it, they could simply be left alone, continuing to walk along the precipice of madness.

When it came to treatment that worked, the morally insane man of the late nineteenth century would have to wait. The hysterical woman, on the other hand, was about to become patient zero in a treatment revolution—one that would catalyze the modern era of mental illness and health, usher out one name while creating another, and alter modern consciousness forever.

The first spark of that revolution began in 1885 in Paris, where, walking the grounds of the Salpêtrière hospital, a young physician from Vienna saw the forces that had influenced Western medicine laid out before him. Walking through the imposing main entrance, he passed the newly erected bronze statue of Pinel, the great reformer. Beyond that he saw the hospital's seventeenth-century chapel, designed to resemble the Greek cross, a symbol of both antiquity and Christendom.

But the young man, Sigmund Freud, had not come to Salpêtrière for these sights. The main event was found in the hospital's auditorium, once a gunpowder factory under Louis XIII. There he joined an audience of students and physicians who chatted amongst themselves until a hush fell and attention turned intently toward the stage. A woman—the only woman in the auditorium—was seated upon a chair, upright but slack-jawed, as though in a trance. She was, in fact, hypnotized.

The days of Mesmer were long gone. The fall of Emperor Napoleon III in 1870—largely attributed to France's inferior military science in its war with Prussia—had catalyzed a new era of scientific rigor. France had become a leader in medical research and, as part of that trajectory, the undisputed epicenter of the emerging field of psychiatry. The man who most embodied this cutting edge was precisely who Freud had come to Salpêtrière to see—who everyone in the auditorium now looked at as he joined the woman on stage. He was Jean-Martin Charcot, the famed physician and neurologist, known throughout post-imperial France as the "Napoleon of Neurosis." "Neurosis," or "nervous illness," was at this time a term encompassing various conditions hounding medical professionals, including hypochondriasis. Hysteria's inclusion in this group was more controversial—some physicians argued that medicine's greatest mystery should be consigned to a group unto itself, an outlier even among outliers. But it was hysteria that had come to occupy a special place in Charcot's work and career.

Through studying scores of the five thousand women committed at Salpêtrière, Charcot claimed to have brought the wild diagnosis to heel, dismissing the notion that hysteria was an unpredictable, disobedient chameleon. Sanity, he believed, was the product of good heredity and a healthy brain, while insanity was the result of poor heredity and a diseased brain. The hysteric's apparent status between sanity and insanity was only a transient illusion: in fact, she suffered from a degenerative neurological disease that would eventually carry her from one state to the other. (Though Charcot did not present hysteria as a female illness per se, his etiology did not contradict the idea. If one were inclined to see women as inferior to men, it stood to reason that women were especially prone to neurological decay.)

Instead of focusing on the many confusing symptoms with which a hysteria patient could present, Charcot centered the condition on the patient's tendency to dissociate. A term popularized by Charcot's colleague, Pierre Janet, "dissociation" referred to the severing of different psychological domains—such as thought, sensation, speech, memory, and emotion—from one another. Everyone had multiple components to their mental life that needed to work together for experience to make sense—what one saw had to sync up, to some extent, with how one felt and what one thought. Hysterics struggled to maintain this integration, according to both Charcot and Janet, a struggle that could explain any number of symptoms that earlier physicians had found inexplicable. Hysterical blindness, for instance, occurred when visual processing dissociated from the rest of the patient's mind. The problem was not that the patient couldn't see—as in physical blindness—but that she couldn't access the part of her that *could* see with the part of her that had thoughts about what was going on in the outside world.

Charcot presented the ease with which he hypnotized his patients as the ultimate proof that dissociation defined hysteria, concluding in an impressive feat of circular logic that hysteria could be diagnosed based solely on whether a person could be hypnotized. Though Charcot had made little progress toward treatment, or shown much interest in it, doctors across Europe seemed rapt by the idea that one could diagnose a patient without ever needing to ask her what she was thinking or how she felt.

Now, Charcot walked to the woman in the chair.[34]

"When you wake," he said to her, "you will be unable to use your left arm."

He clapped, the sound echoed through the silent chamber, and the woman seemed to wake. She looked around nervously, perhaps put off by the large audience. Charcot asked her to raise her left arm.

"Oh, but I can't," she replied in a meek voice, and indeed her limb hung at her side as if paralyzed.

"Why not?" the Frenchman asked.

"I don't know . . . perhaps I injured it."

Charcot turned to the audience. "You see, gentlemen, the act of suggestion has removed the patient's ability to operate the arm from consciousness. Not only that. The patient cannot access the suggestion, either, for it was administered during the hypnotized state, which is also dissociated. Therefore, she attempts to explain the symptom using the remaining conscious faculties at her disposal."

As Charcot began again to hypnotize the woman in order to reverse the paralysis, Freud's mind whirred. The performance had riveted him, yet beneath his awe lay a seed of discontent.

The young man from Vienna was not then well known to anyone in the audience, or anyone in the field of medicine at large. At twenty-nine, being a physician was only the latest of his professional endeavors, all of which had, so far, amounted to little. Certainly no one in the room could have known that this man represented a convergence of the disparate, broken lines of hysteria's past and would become the undisputed architect of its future. He was fascinated by the myths and philosophies of antiquity; he despised the tyranny of the Catholic Church; as a secular Jew, he had a personal investment in helping the oppressed and underserved; as a man planning to marry, he was in desperate need of a career that would earn money.

Perhaps above all, Freud wanted to make a name for himself. As a university student of zoology he had dreamt of answering "the eel question," a riddle of animal reproduction that had baffled scientists for centuries; as a budding neuroanatomist he had hoped to crack the mysteries of the brain, to identify the nature of gray matter down to its irreducible parts—not just what the brain was but *why* and *how*.[35] Now the new field of psychiatry called to him, and one aspect in particular. Hysteria, the greatest mystery of the medical world since the dawn of time.

Freud didn't just want to shuttle it from one side of the split to the other. He wanted to understand hysteria, and through that understanding find the answer that had eluded even the Napoleon of Neurosis: how to treat it.

3

PSYCHIC DEATH

Sessions, Weeks 2–19

A na arrived five minutes late to our second session.
"Sorry," she said as she threw herself onto the couch, breathing heavily as though she'd been running. "Lost track of time." Again, she wore all black. She sat facing me—Ana never opted to lie on the couch, and I never suggested she do so—smiling politely as her eyes searched my face for a reaction to her lateness.

I betrayed little. I was feeling calmer than at our last encounter; already I had in mind how the next forty-five minutes would go. First sessions were generally a chance to get acquainted, to hear what bore most prominently on someone's mind, and, in Ana's case, that had steered us toward an intensity I'd barely felt able to contain. But second sessions were when I asked a predetermined set of questions about a patient's past: early family life, school experiences, overviews of past and current employment, medical issues, substance use. At least for today, I would be in control.

"I thought we might take some time to talk about your history," I said.

"My history," Ana repeated with a hint of disgust. "I don't understand. Why do you want to know about that?"

When I dictated to patients the terms of this second session, they usually responded by saying, "Okay." Some expressed relief that, after the ambiguity of the first session, they could rely on me to lead the discussion for a while. No one had ever asked *why*. Doctors needed information and patients needed to provide it. That was just how it worked.

Forced to reflect, I did have reasons. Taking a patient's history gave a bird's-eye view of her experiences and, even more, the stories those experiences helped to create. History is process as much as content; what someone says is given context by how she says it. When I ask, "How would you describe your childhood?," one of my standard inquiries, I am looking less to gather facts (which I could never verify anyway) than to observe the present iteration of a personal narrative, which is fluid and subject to revision. Two patients might report similar "facts" about their early environments—raised by biological parents who held stable jobs in a middle-class suburb, say—but the one who declares, "I never had anything to complain about," is telling a different story than the one who says, "I received a lot of support, but I also clashed with my parents sometimes, especially when I was a teenager."

I explained some version of this rationale to Ana as it occurred to me, and she agreed to answer my questions. She told me she'd grown up as an only child in San Antonio, Texas. Her parents divorced when Ana was six years old.

"How would you describe your childhood?" I asked.

"Fine," she said. "Weird. I don't know. My parents fought all the time. My dad hit her. He socked me in the stomach once. Threw me down the stairs. But I always thought he was cooler, you know. He's smarter than my mom and would buy me things and let me stay up late, stuff like that. I remember one time sneaking a look into their bedroom after a big fight, my mom was sitting on the bed crying and my dad was sitting next to her, fondling her breast." She shuddered and looked at me as though waking from a trance, then laughed nervously. "What was your question?"

Ana didn't have amnesia, the condition of being without memory. But she seemed to lack a *history*, a narrative that would give her memories meaning: the understanding of cause and effect, of why something happened in the way it did, how it made her feel, and how those circumstances and feelings informed what happened next. The patient who said she'd had "nothing to complain about" as a child might be spinning an oversimplified yarn, but at least it was stable. For such a patient, anytime the notion came up that her early experience might be exerting its influence on her present-day life, she could turn the autobiography in her mind back to the first chapter and reject the offending notion: *No, that cannot be, I had nothing to complain about.* Psychotherapy with such a patient would involve the gradual expansion of that inner text, taking a clean but impoverished narrative and fleshing it out. Ana, by contrast, seemed to be seeing something different every time she flipped back the pages of her memory: was she hero or villain, victim or aggressor? Her life story was like a jumble of scenes from a heavily redacted novel, roughly in order but stripped of the guiding language needed to follow the plot.

"Wait, how did you end up in the hospital?" I asked after Ana described an episode in which she'd gotten drunk at school at age fourteen, attacked a teacher, and spat on the police officer who had arrived on the scene.

She paused and glanced to the side, brow furrowed. I recognized that look from my undergraduate years in writing workshops: the look of a writer realizing she's the last to know her story doesn't make sense.

"Oh, yeah," she said. "I guess I started screaming that I was going to kill myself."

Surprise and contradiction lurked around every corner. Ana spoke of how close she was to her family, especially her father, but also said she had fled Texas for New York in order to escape them. She swung from tears to laughter to a striking aloofness, seemingly without regard for what was being discussed, as though her thoughts and emotions operated independently of one another. It was hard to keep straight which aspects of her experience were over and which were ongoing. She apologized at multiple points for not knowing certain dates or having gaps in her timeline. "I feel like the last five or six years I've been able to access less and less from my past," she said. She admitted she wasn't sleeping much these days. She had resumed referring to Tom as her ex.

At the end of the session I asked Ana how it had been to talk through her history in this way. She said it had made her "anxious," a word I would learn could serve for her as proxy for a range of feelings that, for the time being, she could not otherwise describe.

"I'm embarrassed by how emotional I've been. I don't want you to think my childhood or family were all bad."

"I don't think that," I said. "But it sounds like your early life was very chaotic."

"That's probably why I like stimulants so much. They help me tune out the noise. My favorite thing to do right now is take Adderall and read books."

It was time to stop. Ana asked if meeting more than once a week was something I ever did with patients. I said it was, and we agreed to meet later in the week to see how that felt to her.

"Oh, and I've decided I'm going to pay for this myself," she said. We were using the insurance she received through her job as a cashier, which left a modest copay per session. Tom's promise of financial support, it turned out, had been more symbolic than necessary.

"I think that makes sense," I said.

"I've had that debit card for years, you know. The one with the wolf on it. I'd never thought about why before. You showed me something I didn't know was there."

And she left.

The gravity in her voice as she said those last words unnerved me. What had I shown her? I strained to remember what I had said the week before. *Oh God*, I thought. *She's really listening to me.*

———

The following week Ana sat down and pulled a bag of Peanut M&M's out of her purse. She opened it and began to eat with conviction, staring fixedly ahead, as though the nut hidden in each candy contained an idea and with each bite she expanded her capacity to think.

She said she had a lot on her mind. She'd composed five or six long emails to me the night before but sent none of them, feeling unsure of the "rules" around contacting me outside of our scheduled sessions. Before I could respond to this she continued, saying she still wasn't sleeping much, that she enjoyed being up when it felt like the rest of the city was not, or perhaps she was scared to sleep, she wasn't sure, and in the meantime she'd been reading a lot. *A lot.* Although we hadn't discussed theory directly, she said she presumed, based on the information on my website, that I was familiar with Sigmund Freud and some other psychoanalysts she had been reading. But did I know much about Descartes?

"I think they have a lot to say to each other," she said.

I recalled the Adderall comment Ana had made the other day and got lost in my own thoughts on how to assess if she was high right now, and whether I would feel comfortable asking her outright.

"Also, I did a stupid thing last night," she said. "I went to Tom's apartment and tried to force him to have sex with me. That was probably a mistake."

"Okay," I said. In an instant I could see Ana's energy fading. She became tearful and seemed to shrink in stature. I ventured, "You're feeling ashamed?"

"Yes. I thought if I could convince him . . . that, if we could recreate the scene, but this time I was directing it. . . . Now, I'm so confused. Would someone who was actually raped do something like that?"

What Ana described was, in a sense, Freud's repetition compulsion, something she had not yet come across in her frenzied readings.[1] The theory goes that we're driven to recreate that which has overpowered us in the past, to prove to ourselves that we have mastered its conditions. This drive operates without—and sometimes directly against—conscious intent, and often serves to re-traumatize or pass trauma on to others. A father who was beaten as a child may take a fist to his own son, in part, to denigrate his own abuse, to prove that it held no power then and holds no power now, and thus leaves the child to carry the burden forward. Ana had literalized the process and sped it up: within weeks of being raped she had returned to Tom and begged him to rape her again. She wanted to negate the first trauma by claiming ownership over the second. Tom had apparently filmed her pleas on his phone and then kicked her out of the apartment.

I attempted a clumsy explanation of the repetition compulsion, landing on the point that Ana's recent actions could not undo her past suffering. On one hand this was unfortunate, I said, because it meant the rape could never be taken back. But it could also be a stabilizing idea, that this part of her story would not change—no matter what she did now, the rape would still have happened and it would still not be her fault. As painful as that piece of her history was, it could be relied upon.

Ana nodded. "There's something I haven't told you," she said. "The dream I had, the one that convinced me to see a therapist, to see you. . . . It's true that in the dream I was visited by a spirit, a woman I didn't recognize but felt that I knew, and it's true she told me that I was a descendant of abuse. That being raped was inevitable and maybe not a bad thing to the extent that it connected me to those who came before. But that's not all she told me." Here, Ana paused and glanced at me, smiling a strange, nervous smile. "She said that part of the dowry—if you can call it that; well, that's what she called it—was my death. That, in fact, the rape had killed me and I was dead. I mean, I *am* dead. So, you're treating a corpse, which maybe is a first for you."

As in our very first session, Ana's balletic leaps from eloquence to incoherence to gallows humor left me stunned, as if in awe, unsure of what to call the thing I had just experienced.

"To be sure I understand," I said, as though I were just one clarifying question away from a state of knowing, "you *feel* like you're dead, or you believe that you *are* dead?"

Ana looked down and I could sense her disappointment. My question had been diagnostic in the crassest sense; I was "reality testing," a clinical term for gauging not what a patient sees but the extent to which she sees what *I* see. Which, of course, presumed that my own ability to test reality was intact.

"I know I'm not dead like a body in the graveyard is dead. I walk, I talk, I eat food. I'm here, aren't I?"

"Yes, I see and hear you, and you look alive to me."

"Have you heard of ego death? I'm not making this stuff up. It's possible to die in stages. My body is still alive but I am dead, not metaphorically dead but *dead* dead. As in, not coming back. Psychic worm food."

I knew the term "ego death"—alternately called "ego loss" or "psychic death," denoting the disintegration of one's sense of being an individual—from cursory readings of Carl Jung and an even vaguer awareness of the psychedelic literature of Timothy Leary.[2] My understanding was that those who wrote about the loss of self in this way viewed it as something to aspire to, a form of transcendence that freed us from the prison of the mind and connected us to Jung's idea of the collective unconscious, or what Leary called the "post-terrestrial."

Ana, I would soon learn, had arrived at a more idiosyncratic definition, derived by her kinetic approach to consuming information: pinging from one idea to the next; ten pages into a dozen books, of which she would finish none; a hundred tabs open on her internet browser. Somewhere along the way, Ana had connected the term "ego death"—the phrasing of which felt to her a perfect match for what was happening internally—with the twentieth-century French psychoanalyst Jacques Lacan, who had never actually used it. It wasn't hard to see how Ana had hop-skipped from one concept to the other. "Ego death," when put into Google, quickly brought up results on the "death drive," a distinct Freudian concept that many writers have grappled with over the last hundred years, including Lacan, who in turn was cited frequently by the contemporary philosopher Slavoj Žižek.[3] When Ana, at the end of this internet rabbit hole, encountered a provocative essay in which Žižek contended that all women harbor rape fantasies, it seemed to her a validation that her own rape had been predestined, and reading the essay had no doubt helped to accelerate her return to Tom's apartment.[4]

"The good news about being dead is that I can't be raped again," Ana said. "What happens to my body doesn't matter anymore." She mentioned that she had slept with a few men recently, all of whom knew she had been raped weeks earlier. These men—each connected in some way to the anarchic party scene Ana had been ensconced in since arriving in New York the previous year—had listened to her "rant" for an hour or two, usually after running into Ana at a music show or bar. She saw sex as recompense for their attention.

"So, just by speaking to someone about what you're going through, you accrue a debt that must be repaid?" I asked.

For perhaps the first time, Ana corrected me: the process was not transactional but metabolic. "Sex is like taking a shit after a big meal," she said flatly. "I fill them up with my thoughts and they put the garbage they don't want back into me at the end."

I said nothing. Years later Ana would tell me that the look on my face in such moments helped her, more than anything I ever said, to see how far she was from herself.

"Do you have a plan?" Ana asked me about a month into our treatment. "What is the goal here? Where are you taking me?"

It had been apparent to me for some time that Ana met criteria for BPD as it appeared in psychiatric manuals, and more or less as I understood it from my training in psychoanalytic theory. Though I had worked with people already carrying the mark of BPD, I'd not yet wielded the brand myself—and holding an idea about a person is not the same as sharing it with her. Diagnosis is always a delicate process, and I felt a special weight when it came to a patient who seemed prone to losing herself in the gaze of others. Should I diagnose someone who might not be in a state of mind to advocate for herself—that is, to disagree if she felt I was off the mark? But by the same token, didn't I owe it to Ana to tell her more about what she was going through if I possessed that knowledge?

Now seemed as good a time as any to discuss a formal diagnosis. Ana trembled when I mentioned the idea. "I don't trust labels," she said. "But I also feel like you're the first doctor I've met whose label I might trust."

"I think you have borderline personality disorder," I said. "Have you heard that term before?"

"Yes," she said. She paused, became tearful, and smiled. "Great. So, I'm a psychotic basket case." She described a couple of women she had met in the past who'd said they had BPD, how unstable and needy they were. The exact word she used was "hysterical."

I emphasized the aspects of BPD that I thought would resonate with Ana: the pervasive feelings of emptiness; the use of splitting to organize her views of herself and others; the tendency toward impulsive, often self-destructive action when faced with overwhelming emotion. I said the condition as I understood it was connected to chronic experiences of trauma or abuse starting from an early age. It did not represent the totality of who Ana was, but the part of her that had been forced to deal with unusually difficult circumstances.

At the end of the session, Ana appeared visibly shaken. "I probably shouldn't research this when I go home," she said.

I agreed. BPD was a fraught term, I said, but I'd introduced it into our therapy because we needed common language to help Ana define her experience. Saying she had "anxiety" wasn't going to cut it, even if that word was more socially acceptable than "borderline"—in fact, using "anxiety" or any other inadequate label would mislead Ana about the nature of her suffering and how it might best be treated.

After Ana left, I spent the rest of the afternoon wondering if what I'd just set in motion was an honest, ethical discharge of my professional duty, or a big mistake.

"I found something out about you," Ana said in the middle of a session, about two weeks later. The comment seemed apropos of nothing. We had been talking about Ana's difficulty sleeping after she'd seen a post Tom had made on Facebook in which he described himself as a feminist.

"Oh?" I said.

"Yes, and I think I hate you now."

"We should probably talk about that."

"I know who your father is!" she declared, too loud and with a finger pointed to the ceiling, as though she were a private detective calling out the killer among suspects gathered in a Victorian parlor.

I knew immediately what she meant. Ana's gifts as an internet spelunker were already established, and finding my father's name was certainly within her means. And once she found his name, she would have found the photograph.

"Ah," I said. "Maybe you do."

Ana held her tense posture, waiting for more. When nothing came, she relaxed slightly; her hand returned to her lap.

"Why aren't you more shocked?" she asked. "This is anticlimactic."

"I'm not shocked that you googled me. A lot of patients do, I think. Maybe you dug deeper than most, but that doesn't shock me either. I am interested to know why you feel you hate me now."

Ana appeared deflated; the "gotcha" moment had passed. As this settled in, a new anger began to rise, something pricklier.

"Because you're a child of privilege raised by a capitalist pig," she said. "So, tell me, do you do this work as penance, or do you get off on emotionally exploiting people from a position of power?"

About the photograph. In 1984 my father and a handful of colleagues at a new Boston-based venture capital firm held a photo shoot to create a promotional brochure. After a while, my father made a suggestion: why not take a gag shot, just for the group, in which everyone is flashing a bunch of cash? The photograph likely would have remained largely unseen had one of the seven men in it not been Mitt Romney, 2012 Republican nominee for president of the United States. On October 13, 2011, less than a month to Election Day, it was published on *The Atlantic*'s website with the title, "Picture of the Day: Mitt Romney's Money Shot."[5]

I was in graduate school at the time. I had never seen the photograph before, and was still grappling with how to integrate privilege into my understanding of my life and history. I'd tried hiding it, acting like I knew what college friends were talking about when they spoke of their debts. I'd tried denying it, telling myself that any good fortune I enjoyed was reparation for the suffering of my Jewish ancestors. On the phone with my father, he said that several journalists had called him for a comment about the photograph, but he'd declined them all.

I couldn't believe it. This was so embarrassing, I said. Didn't he want to explain himself?

The photo was dumb, he agreed. But why try to defend it? It was meant to be private and now it was public. It was meant to be a joke and now no one found it funny. It was embarrassing, yes, in the way that looking back at your younger self—the brashness, the self-importance, the ambition—is often embarrassing.

"But people don't see it as a time capsule of younger selves," I said. "They're saying this is indicative of who you all are."

There was silence on the line. "Well, that's very sad," my father said. "If I'm the same person now as I was then, what was the point of the last twenty-seven years?"

"Are those my only options?" I asked Ana. "Savior or sadist?"

She looked at me with a mix of annoyance and surprise. Another anticlimax.

"You found a photo of my father on the internet," I went on, "and you want to believe that photo tells you all you need to know about me. But the truth is we're still getting to know each other. You won't come to know me from what you find out there. It will come from how I treat you in here."

I'd had to fight a strong pull to defend myself to Ana. To prove my worth and good intentions in the face of her apparent judgment. But to what end? I didn't agree with her assessment of me or my family, but was it so intolerable for me to hear it that I needed to abandon my responsibility as her therapist in order to become my own apologist? Or, perhaps the pull came more from a part of me that wanted to give Ana what she seemed to be looking for: a fight. She saw me as something powerful but dormant, a sleeping leviathan, so she unconsciously poked at me, simultaneously hoping and fearing that doing so would wake me up and cause me to attack.

"I don't really hate you," Ana said. "I thought I did, but I don't feel it anymore. I *do* worry about why someone becomes a therapist. Do you feel things? Can you be a whole person? And just now, did you trick me into not hating you anymore, or can I trust that it's real?"

"You don't have to answer those questions today," I said. "That urge to know, to deny uncertainty and act on half-formed thoughts— what we might call impulse—is something you can learn to sit with."

The conversation left an impression. Whatever Ana thought she knew about me and my history, she had to admit that she never felt unsafe in my presence. My patience with her distrust of authority helped—as did my refusal to lash out when provoked—but more than anything she responded to my commitment to being myself. When she tried to define me I didn't chastise her, but I also didn't lose myself in her reality by turning aggressive, becoming the monster she felt compelled to expose. Even when Ana laughed and called me a "therapy-bot," even when she raged that I was too unfeeling, my consistency felt like something stable she could grasp amid the squall of her daily life. She could throw at me whatever she needed to throw; she could say whatever was on her mind. It wouldn't change me. It wouldn't end our relationship.

Inside, I was hardly Galen's model of a dispassionate therapist. Remaining myself felt less like standing on solid ground than fighting to maintain an illusion of stillness during an earthquake. Sometimes I would find myself quivering in my office before our session, forcing myself to eat a sandwich during the brief lunch break I allotted myself despite feeling nauseous. Was I coming down with something? Then Ana and I would meet, she would leave, and my body would feel at rest again. I had been nervous to see her.

For a while I didn't admit this to myself—to think that a part of me dreaded sitting with Ana felt like a betrayal of her newly earned sense of safety. But this shift was inevitable: as Ana felt calmer in my presence, I felt her pain more acutely. She carried her pain with her everywhere, trying to survive each day with an abusive ex-boyfriend (who continued to lord over her from afar with threats of posting online the video in which she begged to be raped), unsupportive friends (several of whom were, more accurately, sexual predators), and difficulty performing at work, all while living in a traumatized mental state.

In her literalist mindset—where she could not fully distinguish feeling dead from being dead—Ana interpreted the newfound sense of peace that our relationship brought as belonging to the physical space of my office. I noticed that she would grip the arm of the couch fiercely when she first sat down and again as she prepared to leave, like she was about to step out of a capsule into the void of space. One day I commented on this. She smiled sheepishly and looked around the room.

"I do sometimes think I would like to stay," she said.

"What do you mean?"

"It's chaos out there. Sometimes I walk around for hours, but I can't seem to come back to how I feel when I'm here. So, sometimes I think I'd like to stay." She laughed in the way one does when trying not to cry. "I could just tuck myself away . . . you wouldn't even know I was here. If another patient asked, you could say, 'Oh, that's just the girl under the couch!'"

At the start of our fourth month of treatment, Ana and I began to meet four times a week. She knew something real was happening, between us and inside of her, but she had little context with which to understand it. Despite her modern education and feminist inclinations, Ana identified with the ancient notion of her female mind and body being inflamed and out of control. Even if I didn't feel it myself, to her I was Galen's preternaturally calm man, the boron rod that could temper her radioactivity just by being physically close.

One Sunday afternoon she sent me an email, breaking the seal off the prohibition she had imposed on herself not to contact me outside of our sessions.

Dr. Kriss,

I decided to sit with my impulses and it has been extremely difficult, but I'm doing it and I feel very proud of myself. The first major impulse that I restrained gave me a triumphant feeling and the rest have been like aftershocks.

I really understand those impulses now . . . what they were protecting. Giving myself the space to think has allowed me to accept Tom for who he is, the choices he made, and that I can't force him to be accountable or love me. I finally made the choice to let him go, I wrote him a goodbye letter, and of course he's blocked me from everywhere so I can't give it to him. I'm still getting strong impulses to find a way to reach him, to command power, but I know there's no point. Even if he read it, it wouldn't mean anything anyway. There is no purpose to this evil.

But now I'm in tremendous grief . . . more than I could have expected. I haven't been able to leave my room for days and I can't stop crying. It's not depression because I don't want to die, it's just pain, I just feel so sad . . . I almost forget what I'm crying about sometimes.

I tried to read but that didn't work. It's like the writers have stopped speaking to me and it's gibberish now. Zizek is a pig. So, I put away all the books, all the distractions, and tried to trick myself into thinking I was doing some noble intellectual meditation like Descartes . . . . when he would isolate himself for hours in silence to just Think. The sad, boring truth is that none of this is noble or glorious, it's just the same shit we all feel.

So, should I sit with this grief or should I distract myself? Should I start to think about ways to punish Tom or should I wait? It still feels unfair that he can live without feeling the consequences of his actions. Should I go out and party or try to forget? I can't decide . . .

Every session with you is easy to get through and then I'm destroyed afterwards.

—Ana

Ana felt caught between worlds. The wordless, prehistoric dynamic of a wolf devouring its prey no longer captured her experience, but neither did modern intellectual discourse—from Žižek's twenty-first-century philosophy of rape all the way back to René Descartes's 1641 *Meditations on First Philosophy*, the titans of the Western canon all failed to meet Ana where she was.

In the weeks following her email, Ana found a new fascination: the history of witches and witchcraft. It was a worldview that made sense to her: the merciless persecution of women, the split of good and evil. Disturbing questions of her role in her own rape, which had hounded her at the start of our meetings, calcified into the idea that Tom was simply an evil man who had committed an evil act. At long last, here was a story Ana could use to begin writing her history. It was one of the oldest stories in human culture: the battle of light versus dark. She started avoiding her old group of friends, especially the men who had taken advantage of her sexually, compelled by the notion that they were in league with Tom, that they were his demonic minions.

The cost of this split was any sense of nuance. If there was only good and evil, then someone was always abusing and someone was always being abused. This posed a particular complication for our relationship, which had come to feel like such a reliably safe space for Ana. The feeling that my office was a port in her life's perpetual storm gave way to a belief that she had successfully fooled me into thinking she was a likable human being, when in fact she was something else, something worse.

One night I received a voicemail from Ana in a state of abject anxiety. She stuttered and repeated herself, and at points shouted syllables I couldn't understand.

"S-s-s-see?" she ended her message. "This is what I'm r-r-really like. I'm not g-g-g-good."

It was unclear if by "good" Ana was speaking in terms of her mental health or mortal soul; I don't think she was at that time distinguishing between the two. In session she began referring to herself with a knowing smile as "the Devil's midwife," an inscrutable moniker derived from a book she had half-read (before becoming overwhelmed and burying it beneath a pile of clothes in her closet) about how midwifery was considered heretical during the Dark Ages. But I also think she meant to communicate her sense of carrying the Devil's child. A feeling that, after her rape, a darkness had formed within her that could never be purified. This feeling of inner rottenness gradually replaced Ana's belief that she had died.

"I don't need a therapist," she told me at one point. "I need an exorcist."

She wondered if the spirit from her dream had actually been a demon in disguise, and that everything that followed—including meeting me—was a cruel trick, another step in the endless path of her damnation.

4

SEDUCTION AND FANTASY

1896–1923

"Imagine that an explorer arrives in a little-known region where his interest is aroused by an expanse of ruins, with remains of walls, fragments of columns, and tablets with half-effaced and unreadable inscriptions," Sigmund Freud said before the Vienna Psychiatric Society on April 21, 1896, eleven years after watching Charcot's performance at Salpêtrière. "He may content himself with inspecting what lies exposed to view, with questioning the inhabitants—perhaps semi-barbaric people—who live in the vicinity, about what tradition tells them of the history and meaning of these archaeological remains, and with noting down what they tell him—and he may then proceed on his journey."

He surveyed the crowd of primly dressed men, gleaning little from the unmoving faces obscured behind a haze of cigar smoke.

"But he may act differently," Freud continued. "He may have brought picks, shovels and spades with him, and he may set the inhabitants to work with these implements. Together with them he may start upon the ruins, clear away the rubbish, and, beginning from the visible remains, uncover what is buried."[1]

The revolution was underway.

It may not appear so: Freud's haute speech, suffused with colonial imagery, may seem exactly the sort of thing a roomful of white, male doctors would be chattering about in a Viennese parlor at the turn of the twentieth century. But, as Freud and his colleague Josef Breuer had begun writing about in the preceding years, appearances could be deceiving.

First, in the eyes of the crowd, Freud was not white—at least not by the modern implication of that word, denoting membership to the most privileged and free group within a racial hierarchy. Universities under the Austro-Hungarian Empire had only begun admitting Jews in the 1860s, and they were relegated to what the gentile majority regarded as lesser fields, including psychiatry.[2] Even then, Freud would have been one of the only Jewish men in the room as he stood before the Society, the most prestigious psychiatric organization in Vienna. A Jewish man was, in fact, far more likely to be treated for hysteria than to be the one treating it: records from nervous clinics of the era show that Jews and women were often grouped together diagnostically, segregated from the labels afforded to Christian men.[3]

Second, if one suspected Freud of feeding the old boys their usual tripe, the silence that followed his presentation, which he called "The Etiology of Hysteria," said otherwise. "The asses gave it an icy reception," Freud would later write to his friend Wilhelm Fliess.[4] Instead of the usual applause and compliments, members urged Freud to leave his work unpublished. The chair of the Society, an eminent psychiatrist named Richard von Krafft-Ebing, dismissed Freud's central concept as a "scientific fairy tale." That central concept was a radical view of hysteria that defied all conventional knowledge that preceded it: it defied Sydenham's emphasis on observable symptoms as the targets of treatment, it defied Charcot and Janet's insistence on the primary role of heredity, it defied even Descartes's centuries-old segregation of body and mind.

Freud loved metaphors, and over his career would employ many of them—steam hydraulics to describe the pressure and release of sexual drives; an army garrison to represent our internalization of the strictures of civilization—but the foundational metaphor of psychoanalysis was the one he laid out in his 1896 speech: the archaeological expedition.[5] The "semi-barbaric people" were the hysterical patient's conscious mind, living without history, severed from the lineage of past experience that would explain present problems. Psychoanalysis would be the reclamation of that lineage, the search for truth beneath the surface.

The suggestion in this metaphor that the explorer knows best—that a foreign archaeologist is better equipped to discover truth on native land than the natives themselves—encapsulates the radical-conservative tension that would define Freud's career and global influence. Women represented, of course, the bulk of the patients Freud was attempting to understand when he turned his attention to hysteria, and his description of them as "semi-barbaric" was consistent with how he considered them in general: inferior, belonging in domestic roles that supported the intellectual, patriarchal bourgeois society of Freud's day. But the metaphor was also an indictment of how physicians—the men he was speaking to—dealt with hysterics. Their only aim, it seemed to Freud, was to resolve symptoms to the patient's immediate satisfaction—or, more often, to the satisfaction of the husband or father who had brought her in for treatment—regardless of whether it actually got to the root of the problem. If a patient was overly excitable, she was given a sedative; if she was overly sedate, she was subjected to electric shocks or ice baths to activate her body. If symptoms went away, she was declared "cured"; when they returned, the same ineffective treatments were trotted out again.

In other words, Freud saw that doctors relied solely on the patient's self-report and external symptoms—those weather-worn artifacts visible on the surface—to guide their actions. It was absurd, Freud said, for a physician to expect a patient to understand her own illness well enough to dictate its treatment. Wasn't that why she'd come to the doctor in the first place?

Beneath the surface, Freud said, lay hysteria's etiology. The doctor was needed, desperately, because it was an etiology from which the patient had been disconnected. It had been buried and repressed, its nature deemed unacceptable to the conscious mind, to the people living above ground. Here the radical Freud emerged, confident and unapologetic before a deeply unsympathetic audience, asserting that the patient's mind had been driven to barbarism not because of heredity, or the inferiority of being a woman, but because of trauma. Something terrible had happened to her and, as a means of self-defense, she had been forced to sacrifice self-knowledge. "In every case the memory of earlier experiences," Freud declared, "plays a part in causing the symptom."[6]

Hysteria was itself a metaphor, he went on. Its symptoms were not literal, which was why treating them literally didn't work: they were symbols, "derivatives of memories which are operating unconsciously."[7] This was a revolutionary claim in and of itself, one that Freud and Breuer had proffered in their book, *Studies on Hysteria*, published a year earlier in 1895. But Freud—obsessive seeker of universal truths, as we will see—would not let the matter rest on such vagaries. What good to a doctor was the knowledge that an illness was caused by disowned memories, in the general sense? The memories in question were specific. Hysteria emerged, Freud said, from the repression of memories of sexual abuse.

"Seduction theory," as this claim of Freud's would be known, was based on empirical evidence. Breuer, over the preceding decade, working out of his hospital in Vienna, had been experimenting with a new treatment for hysteria that had yielded a new kind of scientific data: *psychological* data—the thoughts of hysterical patients. Breuer would instruct a patient to speak about one of her symptoms while under hypnosis. He found that she would, eventually, begin to make connections between the symptom and her underlying memories, arriving eventually at what Breuer believed to be her memory of the symptom's first occurrence. Often, as this origin memory was spoken aloud, the patient would be flooded with emotion, followed by a sudden—and, in some cases, lasting—remission of the symptom. The dramatic crescendo of this treatment led Breuer to call it the "cathartic method."[8] It was a method of healing through conversation with another, a revival of the talking cure Galen had invented two thousand years earlier—but now focused on the release, not suppression, of passionate emotion.

No tinctures or pills were required, no leeches or electric shocks—only a doctor inviting a patient to think and speak while in an altered state, and by the 1890s Freud believed that even the altered state was unnecessary. An influential 1886 study by the French physician Hippolyte Bernheim had shown that all sorts of people—men and women alike, including those with no history of nervous illness—could be induced into a hypnotic state, a finding that eviscerated Charcot's long-standing claim that only hysterics could be hypnotized. As Charcot's authority on hysteria rapidly eroded, Freud suggested to Breuer that they jettison hypnotism from their work entirely. Hypnosis didn't distinguish hysterics from anyone else, it risked the patient submitting herself to a doctor's suggestion rather than accessing her actual thoughts, and its use was becoming so distrusted by the medical establishment that their work would never be taken seriously unless an alternative method could be divined.

Freud called this alternative "free association." Rather than inducing a "waking sleep" to get at memories separated from consciousness, the doctor would ask the patient to say aloud whatever came to mind, regardless of its seeming logic or social appropriateness. By teaching a patient to follow her own train of thought—to respect the associative nature of her mind over the internal censors and lifelong conditioning that compelled her to be polite and "make sense"—she would arrive at new thoughts previously held beneath consciousness. This evolution of the cathartic method—which was ultimately named psychoanalysis—would become the premier psychological treatment.

Freud told Society members that, in eighteen cases of Breuer's that he had studied, consisting of six men and twelve women, every one of them featured an association to memories of childhood sexual trauma. Most commonly, the patient had been seduced and abused by a close adult, usually a parent, and usually over a long period of time. In all cases the child over time had pushed these experiences away, disavowed and disintegrated them. And yet they waited in the shadows, erupting years later as hysterical symptoms, "derivatives of memories."

In the years to come Freud would write copiously about the effects of oppressive cultural systems on the individual. He had already shown a radical pessimism when, in *Studies on Hysteria*, he'd written that the goal of treatment was "transforming neurotic misery into ordinary unhappiness."[9] The implication was that individual therapy could not cure societal ills. Yet Freud was not an especial advocate for social reform, either at the time of his 1896 speech or at any other time. His linking of hysteria to sexual abuse was not followed by a call to improve the rights and protections afforded to women and children. Freud wanted to uncover the nature of society more than he wanted to prescribe its betterment. He wanted the etiology, the why, the truth, but demurred from taking a political stand on what to do with that truth once discovered.

Seduction theory did, however, inspire in Freud an understanding of his patients on an individual level—an *empathy*—that would become and remain a hallmark of effective psychotherapy. For the first time in hysteria's history, perhaps the entire history of illness in the West, a practitioner suggested that his colleagues put themselves in their patient's shoes; that they view her symptoms through the lens of her terrifying experience.

"The reaction of hysterics is only apparently exaggerated; it is bound to appear exaggerated to us because we only know a small part of the motives from which it arises," he said in his address to the Society. By discovering what lay beneath the surface, we might not only free the patient from her suffering, but come to see that she is neither weak nor crazy—rather, she is a person forced to adapt to extreme circumstance. Freud concluded, "In reality, this reaction is normal and psychologically understandable."[10] He stepped down from the lectern.

Less than six weeks later he published a paper on his talk, "in defiance of my colleagues," as he wrote to Fliess. Seduction theory deserved, nay demanded, the attention of the psychiatric establishment. Even the objections of Breuer—skeptical that sexual trauma would be found, without exception, at the core of every hysteria case—failed to dissuade Freud any more than Krafft-Ebing's had. How could they, given that Freud believed he'd discovered, as he wrote to Fliess, "the solution of a thousands-years-old problem, a source of the Nile!"[11] This truth would bow to neither friend nor foe, not to the disapproving frowns of gentile doctors nor a faceless Viennese society that chafed at the mention of sexual impropriety. The truth would out; the truth would set us free.

Then, in late September of the following year, Freud quietly turned his back on seduction theory. For the next few years he would discuss it as little as possible, until his new etiology of hysteria was ready to be unveiled, a golden child destined to enjoy far greater influence. For the rest of his life, among voluminous correspondences and published writings, when Freud spoke at all of his original theory, that first child of psychoanalysis, he did so with the penitence of a sinner.

Whether Freud's sin was creating seduction theory or abandoning it depends on who you ask. But in all cases, from his greatest defenders to his sharpest critics, you'll find the answer clouded by the fact that Freud would have loathed the question.

"Let the biographers labor and toil, we won't make it too easy for them,"[12] he wrote to his future wife Martha Bernays in 1885, during the first of several purges in which he set reams of drafts,

diaries, and letters to flame. Most of the primary sources that scholars rely on today, including Freud's letters to Fliess, were saved only
by interlopers who saw posterity as more important than Freud's
wish to cover his tracks. The motivation underlying that wish is a
cause for much debate among the belabored and toiling biographers.
It was a calculated tactic to shield his work from criticism; no, an
unconscious defense against the very thing he helped to invent, that
is, being analyzed; no, a remarkable insight into history's fallibility,
a rejection of the idea that by calling yourself a historian you should
be granted carte blanche to masquerade your biases and embellish-
ments as fact.[13]

The truth, so to speak, cannot be known, but it seems fair to say
that even from the early point of 1885, before the invention of psychoanalysis proper, Freud appreciated the power of narrative. And
he wanted to assure that he would be the sole author of his story.

The more reverent biographers tend to follow the mythology
Freud laid out for them. The real surprise, they say, is not Freud's
abandonment of seduction theory but his adoption of it in the first
place. He pursued, in the early stages of his career, a naive quest
for theoretical parity that led him to believe that specific real-world
events in childhood predicted all cases of an illness as common as
hysteria. This perspective paints Freud as a man willing to learn
from his mistakes. There is truth in this. Freud's ongoing work with
patients played a significant role in his coming to doubt the verac-
ity of seduction theory, as well as its practical usefulness. Between
1896 and 1897, he reported to Fliess multiple dispiriting instances
in which his attempts to steer patients toward repressed memories
of sexual abuse had been counterproductive, causing them to flee
treatment without improvement.[14]

The reverent biographers paint Freud, above all, as a genius.
For the theory that would replace seduction, the one that would
transform Western culture forever, was by Freud's account his and
his alone—the product of his famous "self-analysis" documented
in his 1900 book, *The Interpretation of Dreams*. The thesis of the

"dream book," as Freud called it, can be distilled from the title: dreams had meaning. The internal world that had been dismissed as unknowable since Descartes could not only be known, Freud said, but held explanatory power about human behavior and character. Psychoanalysis was not a scientific fairy tale but a new science of subjectivity, a project to make sense of a part of ourselves, the unconscious, that does not follow the language, laws, or linearity of waking life—in other words, of society. Our dreams, daydreams, even memories—including the repressed memories of hysterical patients—were not literal; they in fact had little or no relation to external reality. They were ciphers of the inner world, and Freud believed he had begun to develop the key to their translation. Specifically, Freud believed that dreams reflected motifs, passed down through generations, that spoke to universal aspects of the human experience. They explained why we behave the way we do, and why society had developed in the way that it had.

Perhaps the most famous motif he identified in the dream book was the one exemplified in the ancient Greek play by Sophocles, *Oedipus Rex*. Freud saw the myth of King Oedipus—who unwittingly murdered his father and married his mother, and in so doing brought pestilence upon himself and all the people of his kingdom, Thebes—as evidence that everyone, for time immemorial, harbored unconscious fantasies of incest. Even more, he claimed, what we call society existed in no small part as a means to tame the incestuous impulse through labeling it as socially destructive—that is, taboo. There was, again, great value in these ideas. Freud identified, in part through acknowledging and writing openly about his own dreams and fantasies, that there was a meaningful distinction to be made between conscious and unconscious desire, and between thought and action. Thinking something was not the same as doing something; fantasizing did not necessarily mean you wanted to bring the fantasy into reality. It stood to reason, then, that remembering something did not necessarily mean the thing had happened.

Memories of sexual abuse in hysteria patients were, according to this new "fantasy theory," the patients' recalling of the ancient myth of Oedipus, recast with modern players. By 1905, in an influential series of essays about childhood sexual development, Freud was describing hysteria's onset in purely internal terms, cut off from any of the external "motives"—that is, acts of sexual abuse—that he had once said were a necessary catalyst. Now, he said, hysteria was a psychic conflict between an "exaggerated sexual craving and excessive aversion to sexuality," the product of an extreme, contradictory inner world in which the individual wanted and feared sex in equal measure, until the only escape became the development of symptoms.[15] The preponderance of hysteria in women—previously explained as the result of girls being disproportionately vulnerable to sexual predation—shifted to a convoluted theory concerning the biological migration of erogenous zones in girls from the clitoris to the vagina throughout the course of puberty.

Why did Freud abandon seduction theory? He wanted to be right, for one thing—to solve the mystery of hysteria once and for all. His self-imposed demand for a universal answer meant that if a single case did not verify seduction theory, he felt compelled to dismiss the entire theory and everything attached to it. Similarly, once fantasy theory was established it had to be validated in every case, no matter the outcome—including its impact, as we will shortly see, on his patients.

Freud also may have underestimated the fortitude it would take to stand behind a theory of widespread sexual abuse. It was disturbing for anyone—no matter how committed to the truth—to consider the implications of seduction theory, not to mention that those implications had the potential to threaten Freud's livelihood, and the existence of psychoanalysis in general. After all, what father would pay for a treatment that, almost by definition, sought to expose him as an abuser?

Some biographers have also suggested that Freud's pivot from seduction to fantasy was less a change of thought than a change of heart—a desire to avoid interrogating his own traumatic memories. Freud's autobiographical writings and letters refer to a childhood marked by various sexual imbroglios and violations: his father's multiple marriages; suspicions of incest between his mother and his half brother; possible hysterical illness in at least one of his sisters; an allusion to his childhood nursemaid acting as his own "teacher in sexual matters."[16] When Freud's father died in October of 1896—"the most important event, the most poignant loss, of a man's life," he later wrote—he began to harbor grave misgivings about promoting a theory that implicated parents as the drivers of disease.[17] The writing of the dream book over the next several years—in which Freud retreated into a self-analysis of his dreams and memories, confronting the myriad taboo desires residing therein—was at least in part a means of processing the grief over his father's death. The end result was the introduction of a new cultural split: between fantasy and reality. For Freud's desired reality—the one in which his father was respectable and absolved of seduction theory's implications—to be kept intact, elements that did not properly conform had to be dissociated to the realm of fantasy.

Between an 1897 letter to Fliess (in which Freud privately confessed to "no longer believe" in seduction theory) and his 1905 papers on sexuality (in which he confidently presented his alternate etiology), two major professional events occurred. One was the publishing of the dream book in early 1900.[18] The other, from October to December of the same year, was Freud's analysis with an eighteen-year-old woman named Ida Bauer.

Better known as "Dora," the pseudonym Freud used in his study, *Fragment of an Analysis of a Case of Hysteria*, Ida came to treatment with classic turn-of-the-century hysteria symptoms: breathlessness, coughing, migraines, periodic mutism, and a sense of pressure on her chest or throat, all with no discernible medical cause, beginning at age seven. She also experienced more idiosyncratic symptoms, such as overwhelming waves of disgust and a "fear of men engaged in amicable conversation."[19] Freud had met Ida once before, in 1898, at which time he had recommended psychological treatment. But when her symptoms spontaneously abated on their own, her father Phillip decided to leave it at that. In 1900, however, Ida wrote her parents a note saying she planned to kill herself; later, she had a blistering argument with her father, fainted, and awoke with no memory of it. Phillip brought Ida back to Freud, though Ida did not want to go, and her father instructed the doctor to "bring her round to a better way of thinking."[20] This directive was not unusual, both in terms of a father setting the terms of satisfactory treatment for his daughter, and in the implication that the treatment should be fast and targeted. Psychoanalysis was, in its initial decades, a short-term and symptom-focused therapy. The goal was to quickly unearth the unconscious material driving specific symptoms, not to understand the whole person—this focus would not significantly change, as we will see, until after Freud's death. For this reason, along with the pragmatic concerns of treatment—Freud and other analysts often had to travel great distances across Europe to meet the growing demand for their services—psychoanalyses in the 1900s and 1910s were typically measured in weeks or months, and almost never in years.

Freud was, when he began treating Dora in 1900, caught between his two theories. Although it had been three years since telling Fliess he'd lost faith in seduction theory, he had suspected since first meeting Ida two years earlier that, in this patient, childhood sexual trauma lay waiting to be unearthed. And he was right: over the course of their early sessions, Ida gradually disclosed a lurid and yearslong history between her and an older family friend, Hans Zellenka. Memories of seduction progressed from the vague and unsettling—Hans sending Ida flowers every day for a year—to the explicit: being forcefully kissed by him at age thirteen and propositioned for sex at sixteen.

Even more destabilizing than the advances was her father's refusal to believe that they had happened. After Hans's proposition, Ida repeatedly tried to persuade her father to cut ties with him and his wife, and Phillip repeatedly denied her requests—he told Freud that his daughter's accusations were "a fantasy that has taken root in her mind."[21] Whether Phillip really believed this or whether he adopted the narrative for selfish reasons—Ida suspected, and Freud believed, that her father was having an affair with Hans's wife—is impossible to determine. But what is clear is how important it was to Ida that Freud believed her. In line with his 1896 talk, he interpreted her symptoms as reactions to the real things that she'd experienced, which was perhaps the first time Ida had ever felt an adult was truly listening. She began to participate in the analysis more freely, disclosing finer details of her life and sharing dreams, which Freud encouraged her to speak about.

But Freud's ability to continue believing Ida came up against his wish to fit her reality to his new fantasy theory. Increasingly, he adopted the position that Ida's illness stemmed from her internal conflict over her taboo fantasy: namely, that, deep down, Ida loved Hans. First, he suggested that the disgust Ida had felt upon being kissed by her seducer as a young teen was evidence of an exaggerated fear of sex, which he now saw as endemic to hysteria—he contended that a "normal" girl would have felt excited, not repulsed, by the advance. Later in the analysis, Freud revised this interpretation by declaring that, in fact, Ida *had* been excited, and it was an involuntary emission from her vagina that had truly disgusted her. Interpretation of Ida's dreams increasingly revolved around how they confirmed her love of Hans; the reality of Hans's behavior, in turn, was increasingly reframed as inert, from a dogged seduction to a more frivolous series of events onto which Ida had projected her desire. Ida's vocal insistence that she did not love but feared Hans was dismissed as resistance; her silent nods to Freud's long musings were taken as a tacit acceptance of the truth.

In what would be their final session, Freud suggested that Ida's most severe symptoms, including her suicidal thoughts, were not so much prompted by Hans's sexual proposition as by her deep regret over telling her parents about it. Ida wished for Hans to proposition her again, wished even for him to leave his wife and, now that she was of age, marry her instead. She was ashamed that her fantasy did not match reality, and her symptoms arose to push this shame from consciousness. "I know now what you don't want to be reminded of," Freud told her. "It is that you imagined he was making advances to you in earnest, and would not desist until you married him."[22]

Confident in his understanding of Ida, Freud struggled in the closing pages of his study to account for what happened next. "She had been listening without, as usual, raising objections," he wrote. "She seemed to be moved, said goodbye in the most charming way, wishing me every happiness in the New Year, left—and did not come back."[23]

Across the various accounts of Freud's life, the word used to describe his treatment of seduction theory is "abandonment." In therapy with borderline patients there often comes a time when an explicit conversation about this word is needed, to make clear that abandonment is a very particular kind of loss. It is loss without warning, without context, and without end; it is traumatic loss, loss that disrupts a fundamental sense of safety, of reality. Once you've known such a loss it can be difficult not to see any loss as an abandonment, as something all-consuming and destabilizing. The death of an ill grandparent, the end of a romantic relationship that wasn't working—even if my patient is the one who ended it—are all crammed into the template of a wound that never heals, that teaches you nothing, that bleeds out forever until there's nothing left inside of you.

The scholars say Freud abandoned seduction theory because that is precisely what he did. His decision to replace it with fantasy theory was done in secret, in a state of shame and grief. Freud ripped out the central idea that seduction theory had affirmed—that the behaviors of hysteria patients were "normal and psychologically understandable" responses to trauma—and he did it so abruptly and completely that it left not only patients but Freud's acolytes, critics, and future biographers wondering what had happened. Following his own repetition compulsion, he recreated the circumstances that perpetuated the disorder he ostensibly was trying to cure: by denying the reality of a patient's lived experience, Freud withheld from her the same coherent history that had been stolen from her as a child. Hysteria was once again a sickness, rather than a reaction to a sick society.

As a result, the history of BPD itself now splits in two. One path is bathed in light: the history of psychoanalysis's meteoric rise, in the course of which, paradoxically, hysteria would recede into shadow. We will first follow that more public, visible path of success embodied by Freud, before considering in chapter 6 the path that ran parallel to it, underground, embodied by his colleague Sándor Ferenczi.

The eventual success of psychoanalysis was incredible given how nearly every aspect of it flew against the prevailing winds of medical authority. Dreams, not bile or brain tissue, were the material to be studied; dream interpretations, not leeches or tubs of cold water, were the treatments to be administered. Most defiantly of all, reason was not humanity's defining characteristic—it was an irrational urge, especially toward the pleasure of sexual gratification, that lay at our core.

Perhaps the most important driver in Freud's ascent was his gift of synthesis. This, like many of the sculptors of human culture before him, was his great genius. Psychoanalysis thrived despite being a countercultural movement because Freud recruited all other contemporary countercultural movements under its banner: neo-romantic philosophers responded to the primacy he gave to emotional experience; Marxist revolutionaries saw in his descriptions of taboo and self-censorship the psychological consequences of capitalism; sexual reformers, anti-asylum reformers, and doctors looking for novel treatments all saw in Freud's theories the promise of progress.

Freud not only gave to these schools of thought but also borrowed from them, and he borrowed as well from his colleagues who made up the initial psychoanalytic cohort: Sándor Ferenczi, Otto Rank, Karl Abraham, Alfred Adler, Carl Jung, and others. The more diverse perspectives Freud incorporated into his thinking, the more his work appealed to a diverse audience. But Freud did not see psychoanalysis as an exchange of these ideas—it was their terminus. The ideas flowed to him, he synthesized them, and then he demanded adherence to his synthesis.

It was a remarkable tightrope to walk, between inclusion and absolute control. Even as Freud used authoritarian techniques—suppressing discord among colleagues; applying threats and social pressure—to maintain a hold over his movement, it would be inaccurate to portray the early decades of mainstream psychoanalysis as wholly oppressive. Freud's drive to see his creation succeed was also suffused by humanitarian ideals and a genuine excitement that he was on to something. In some cases he sought explicitly to throw off the oppressions of the past and undermine medical authority: rather than seek the approval of Vienna Psychiatric Society types, Freud declared that becoming an analyst should not require a medical education at all. All that should be required was being psychoanalyzed yourself. Once you came to know thyself as Freud had (never mind that he had done so alone, sans analyst), once you knew what it *felt* like to be a patient, you were equipped to do the work, regardless of background. Here was a treatment by and for the people. Anyone could become an analyst, and anyone could benefit from being analyzed.

Well, almost anyone. In theory, psychoanalysis sought to eradicate the insanity-sanity split—increasingly described in psychiatric circles in terms of psychosis (suffering that required confinement to an asylum) on one side and neurosis (suffering that could be treated while living free) on the other. Freud had boldly placed himself on a psychotic-neurotic continuum in the dream book, disclosing his own perverse fantasies and declaring such fantasies to be present in all individuals, no matter how "healthy" they appeared to be. But in practice psychoanalysis could not find a place for everyone. Some people, namely those exhibiting more psychotic symptoms, did not seem to improve under analysis. Freud contended this was because those poor souls could not participate in what first-generation analysts came to believe was an essential ingredient to the success of treatment: the transference.

Transference is, essentially, the conscious and unconscious expectations we bring to new relationships. Freud and others noticed, as more data from clinical practice came in, that patients tended to attribute powerful and specific intentions to the analyst, even though much of what the analyst tried to do was direct patients to focus on themselves. One patient might declare that her analyst's instruction to free associate was sadistic, while another bemoaned her feeble mind's inability to adhere to the doctor's sage wisdom. In the face of a unique and ambiguous situation—sitting in a room with a relatively quiet analyst and being asked to speak your thoughts aloud, no matter how strange or inappropriate they may seem—many patients, all patients in fact, seemed to possess a reflex to fill in the gaps, to reach into the templates in their minds and project them onto the situation and person in front of them. Naming what the patient transferred into the therapy relationship was often a more direct route to underlying fantasies than either free association or dream interpretation, the two primary tools of analysis thus far. The analyst could simply observe how the patient was dealing with *him* as a means of unpacking unconscious dynamics and, with them, the source of illness.

Freud ruled out psychosis as an "analyzable" condition because he believed it produced transferences too wild to be of use to the analyst. Patients with psychosis could not attach to an analyst or see him in a stable way, and their distinction between inner and outer realities was often blurred. A neurotic patient might treat the analyst *as though* he were her father, but a psychotic patient might, within the intensity and ambiguity of treatment, become truly confused and, for instance, believe that her doctor *was* her father.

Here arose a new paradox for hysteria, to pile onto the others. On one hand, hysteria had served as the prototypical condition of psychoanalysis, as the starting point for determining what, if anything, could be successfully analyzed. It had also been, since well before psychoanalysis, the vexing link between sanity and insanity, psychosis and neurosis, the chameleon that could as much resemble the complaints of a functioning member of society at the office of an expensive physician as it could the screams of a madwoman confined to bedlam. How could hysteria be the primary subject of analysis if it were capable of veering into territory deemed unanalyzable?

This paradox resolved the same way the others had, and as history demanded it: hysteria changed. Part of the change came about because, for many patients in the poorly understood middle space between neurosis and psychosis, psychoanalysis worked. It worked in the sense that symptoms resolved more completely and enduringly than ever before, meaning fewer women diagnosed with hysteria ended up in asylums. It worked also in the sense that it helped to return these women, once in a state of ceaseless unrest, back to a state of functioning, and so back to their extant place as second-class citizens in European life. These were not witches or lepers, but ill women who could be made well and reintegrated into society without questioning whether it was, in fact, society that had made them ill.

As fewer rooms in asylums were occupied by hysteria patients, hysteria's connection to the psychotic end of a shared psychological spectrum was severed. Increasingly, twentieth-century psychoanalytic writing grouped hysteria with other neurotic conditions like phobias, melancholia, and obsessional anxiety. Hysteria was no longer alone—more than that, it was no longer special. And so, slowly at first and then with astonishing rapidity, it faded away.

Freud, certainly, no longer needed hysteria. By the end of the 1910s he began to move in pursuit of something beyond the treatment of any disorder, toward a comprehensive theory of the human condition. His 1923 paper "The Ego and the Id" not only introduced some of Freud's most recognizable terms—id, ego, and superego—but fundamentally reframed psychoanalysis from a form of therapy to a method of explaining human behavior in all its forms. Freud would go on to write about humor, religion, sexuality, art, and the origins of civilization through the psychoanalytic lens, a colossal undertaking for which he traded his ambition of solving history's greatest medical mystery.

Perhaps Freud left hysteria behind believing the work was finished: that fantasy theory really had lifted the millennia-old cloud hanging over medical authority; that it was time to move on to bigger things. Perhaps he believed what he had written at the end of the case study of Ida Bauer, that her disappearance from treatment was a product of her father Phillip seeking to protect his affair with Hans Zellenka's wife. Or, perhaps, on some level, Freud recognized that he had abandoned Ida. Not simply by ceasing to believe her, but by refusing to consider that she might not perfectly fit into a theory that he had arrived at through analyzing himself. Perhaps this is why, despite writing about Ida's case study immediately after her abrupt departure from treatment, he declined to publish it until 1905—*after* he had published his new etiology of hysteria. Perhaps, above all, Freud realized that he couldn't treat people in the real world and advance a universal theory of fantasy at the same time. Once again, he would have to choose.

The radical-conservative tension within Freud would not abate; he was, for the rest of his life, to be defined by this contradiction. He sought truth, yet obscured his own. He exposed the oppressive effect of mainstream society on individuals, yet wanted to become mainstream himself. He showed vulnerability, publishing his dreams and fantasies—even his failed treatments—for the world to see, yet he also insisted that his personal experiences were universal, refusing to consider the uniqueness of his own (or anyone's) psychology or history. Freud reacted fiercely to any criticism that even hinted that his ideas were products of his idiosyncrasies—he refused to be seen as anything but objective. He had watched the downfall of former idols like Charcot, and he knew the perpetual risk of dismissal he faced simply by being a Jew. Freud's life was filled with the inconsistencies and defenses that arose from the warring factions inside himself: on one hand, the desire to be an infallible authority while, on the other, advancing a theory of the mind that declared such a thing to be impossible.

And yet Freud was right—brilliantly right—in distinguishing psychological truth from historical fact. It is now well documented that memories of sexual abuse can be manufactured under certain conditions—such as through the heavy suggestion of an authority figure, like a doctor—which was not known when Freud developed and shared his seduction theory.[24] That first attempt to identify the cause of hysteria was undoubtedly too literal; there needed to be room for fantasy, the inner world of the patient. Everything that happens to us passes through the prism of the mind, and we cannot apply Newtonian laws of cause and effect to that most nonlinear place.

Trauma is not so much an event that happens to us as it is our reaction to that event. It's what we call the disruption of our established reality, an event that breaks the rules we've come to expect our environments to follow—just as hysteria broke the rules of medical authority over and over again—and forces us to reconsider the most basic aspects of what it means to be. Trauma inhibits our ability to connect inner and outer worlds—the events that happen and the memories we create from those events—into a coherent history. Freud understood better than most the importance of autobiography, of creating one's own narrative, so much so that he took pains to thwart those who would attempt to tell his story for him. But in moving from one extreme to another—from a theory of traumatic reality to a theory of fantasy—Freud inhibited the patient's right to tell her story. She would have to fit it through *his* prism.

Freud did the world a great service by dragging the murky unconscious into the light, and a great disservice by burying reality in darkness. As psychoanalysis grew over the first quarter of the twentieth century, it came to see the mind as a prison of subjectivity, where love and hate had no external antecedents, where symptoms were a reaction to internal conflict only, a compromise to find gratification while fending off thoughts of the taboo. It no longer mattered whether the taboo was wetting the bed or being raped in it.

5

FEARS

Sessions, Months 6–10

"I'm standing on the subway platform," Ana said over the phone, crying.

We were scheduled to meet in an hour's time. When I'd answered the phone, I had assumed Ana was calling to say she was running late from work. Instead, she told me she'd been fired.

We were nearing the six-month anniversary of our therapy, and I had come to appreciate that Ana often condensed multiple meanings into a single phrase or gesture that could, to someone who didn't know her, seem provocative. On the phone, I could perceive a dizzying array of thoughts racing through her mind. Without her job, she would lose her insurance, and without her insurance she wouldn't be able to afford therapy. Should she still board the train that would deliver her to my office? Should she throw herself onto the tracks? For the moment all she knew was this: she was standing on the platform.

I told her to come in, that we would figure something out. When Ana arrived she was no longer tearful. She collapsed onto the couch as though pushed, rifled through her purse until she produced the familiar bag of Peanut M&M's, and began to eat.

"Well, I guess this is it."

"Let's slow down for a second. When does your insurance run out?"

"I don't know. The end of the month, I think my boss said. My ex-boss. She was crying when she told me. Isn't that weird? *She* was crying. She said she knows I'm a good person and cares about me but my behavior's gotten so bad, showing up late, missing shifts, blah, blah, blah. I wanted to shout, 'I was raped!' I thought about taking the lipsticks we keep near the register and just going around using them to write on all the walls and mirrors, crazy shit, like, 'We heart rapists,' or, 'Fuck women.'"

"Why didn't you?"

"Honestly, I thought of how ashamed I'd be to tell *you*. That seems messed up to me. Did I control myself or are you controlling me? Why shouldn't I trash this stupid fucking store that doesn't care that I'm barely keeping it together? This isn't therapy, it's brainwashing. . . . I'm sorry, I don't know what I'm saying."

"You lost your job. It makes sense that you'd feel upset."

"I don't care about the job. Fuck money. Fuck rent, I've been homeless before. I'm kidding. Not about being homeless, I've been homeless. But I'm not just going to stop paying rent . . ."

"You've never mentioned being homeless before."

"Oh, really? I guess I'm ashamed of that, too. It was in my early twenties, for a little over a year. I try not to think about it. My roommate's boyfriend was talking the other night about how he used to live out of his car. He spoke with such pride, like he'd earned his poverty bona fides. He said something like, 'You can't really know yourself until you go through an experience like that.' It was gross. I physically wanted to retch. And I thought, 'You *chose* to live in your car.' That's different. I had no choice, I had nowhere to go, I'd been turned away by everyone and was fucking broke. But again I didn't say it, and again it's because of you! And that's the sick truth: I don't care about my job or my apartment or my body or my *life*, but I do care about this stupid fucking therapy, and now I can't even have that anymore."

"Nothing dire is happening between us, in this moment. I'm not going anywhere. I'm not just going to disappear. You have insurance until the end of the month. And after that, if needed, we can come to a new arrangement."

"What do you mean? What kind of arrangement?"

"I think it's important that, no matter what, we maintain the basic frame of our relationship. You come here four days a week at a specific time and pay me a specific fee. But if your financial situation has changed, the fee can change."

"To what? I've looked on your website. I can't afford you."

I thought for a moment. "How does five dollars a session sound?"

In the years since, Ana has wondered aloud what direction her life would have taken if I hadn't made this offer. I've wondered the same about my own life. She has asked why I did it, and I've asked myself the same question. There were only so many hours in the week, after all, and I saw Ana for four of them—reducing her fee to virtually nothing had an appreciable impact on the financial position of my practice. I can claim ethics: that my clinical responsibility to Ana at this stage of her treatment exceeded her financial responsibility to me. I can claim privilege: that I, unlike some professionals facing a similar dilemma, could afford to reduce four hours of weekly income. I had substantial cash reserves—mostly money bestowed to me by my parents—a spouse who worked, and, at the time, no dependents.

A big part of my decision was circumstantial: my practice was still pretty new, and I wasn't exactly beating back referrals with a stick. If Ana disappeared from my schedule, four new full-fee patients were not going to take her place. In more recent years, as things have become more hectic, I have been less accommodating with patients whose ability to pay changed, reducing frequency with some or ending treatment altogether with others.

"Not all therapists would do this," Ana said. And it's true—not even I would at a different point in time. A fact made all the more uncomfortable by the effect my decision had on Ana and our relationship. I had subverted an expectation she saw as inviolate: that the instant she could no longer give people what they wanted, they would leave. Subversion is one of the most powerful tools in psychotherapy. It forces us to look around and reflect on the fact that things are not as we assumed they would be.

She continued, "When I was a kid, my therapy with Elaine ended one day and I never saw her again."

"Elaine?" I repeated. "Who's Elaine?"

First homelessness, now this. Fragments of history shaken loose by a tectonic shift, drifting to the surface, or erupting out.

It turned out that Ana had been in therapy for four years as a child at her mother's insistence. Ana couldn't recall what had first brought her there or if she had been given any diagnosis, but she did remember enjoying her weekly afternoon appointments with Elaine. She felt safe there. She felt free to play, or chat, or lie quietly on the couch draped with an embroidered quilt. Then, one day, it just ended. Except, of course, nothing ever just ends. The consequences remain, and the consequences of the consequences. We always add, never subtract.

"I ran away from home," Ana said. "I can't believe I forgot about all this. Or, I guess haven't thought about it for a long time. I was twelve. I convinced my friend from school to go with me, but it was my idea. I can't remember why exactly . . . something about my dad. Anyway, I hated my life. This wasn't like a hide-in-your-friend's-backyard running away. I planned it out weeks in advance, packed a bag, used my dad's credit card to buy bus tickets south. I had this idea that we would head for Mexico.

"We boarded the bus. At first it was exciting. But after a while my friend started getting upset. She seemed to suddenly realize this was really happening. She started crying and somehow we got off the bus . . . I can't remember if they kicked us off or I demanded that the driver stop. Anyway, we wound up at a local police station in the middle of fucking nowhere, all these creepy guys eyeing us as they came through. I remember thinking, 'Oh, anything could happen to me out here.' It hadn't occurred to me before, how dangerous it was.

"They called my dad and he came to pick us up. I think the drive back to San Antonio was at least a couple hours and he didn't say a word. He dropped my friend off and as soon as she left the car he turned around and said, 'I felt like a fool in front of all those cops.' And I burst into tears and apologized, and kept apologizing, but he wouldn't say anything else. He took me straight to my mom's and I think the next day I went to see Elaine. I remember this look on Elaine's face, like she was so disappointed in me. She and my mom talked afterward while I sat in the waiting room. Then in the car my mom told me I wasn't going to see Elaine again, that Elaine was acting like *she* was the mother, that she had kept asking why I had done it, why, why, and it was totally unprofessional. I felt like such a fuckup. I don't think me or my parents talked about Elaine or my running away again."

Up to this point, Ana's father had been evoked in our sessions sporadically, a larger-than-life figure to be feared and admired. Her mother, to my recollection, had only been mentioned twice: once in our second session, when Ana had described the disturbing scene of her father fondling her mother's breast, and again shortly thereafter, when Ana asked if I thought it was weird that her mother had called her up and asked if Ana would consider being a surrogate should she—Ana's mother, a woman in her early fifties—decide to have another child. Yes, I had said, that sounded weird for a number of reasons, not least of which that it's the kind of request one might make of a sister or a friend—not a daughter. "I thought so, too," Ana had said, and her mother disappeared once again into the periphery of the tunnel vision that Ana relied on to navigate the day-to-day assault on her senses.

"I wonder," I said now, "if Elaine was not so much disappointed as concerned."

"Maybe."

"I wonder, also, if the relationship with her ended not because you ruined it by running away, but because your mother felt threatened by that concern."

Ana took a deep breath. "Yes, I could see that." Slowly, she sank deeper and deeper into the couch, her eyes fixed out the window.

"What's going through your mind?" I asked.

"If I position myself just right," she said, "all I can see is the sky, the clouds, and you. Just floating. Totally separate from . . . everything. Like we're not even here on Earth."

"But we *are* here."

"Yes . . . I think I'm in love with you."

She flushed and covered her face with her hands so completely it looked as though she were wearing a mask.

Ana left me a voicemail that evening saying she could never return to my office, she had humiliated herself too thoroughly. But she did return, despite my not especially graceful reaction to her confession of love—I'd said some perfunctory words about how such feelings commonly emerge in treatment, and that discussing them can be an important part of self-discovery. When I next saw Ana she walked her earlier statement back, saying that, actually, she wasn't sure how she felt. And we left it there, a volcano we convinced ourselves would lay dormant—a denial that would, in a few months' time, threaten to destroy our relationship.

Still, Ana did feel more secure in our relationship than any other close bond that had preceded it. Our new financial arrangement suggested that I was not looking for an excuse to abandon her, and from that relative stability Ana felt ready to remember the decades of chaos that had brought her to this point. It was not a conscious readiness, just as none of her memories had been truly forgotten. A part of Ana had been waiting, tirelessly, for a signal to open the floodgates, to release the internal pressure that defined what it meant to live without history, to move from one action to the next on impulse, to lack a continuous sense of herself.

Her emails started pouring in. Some were long and difficult to follow, written in a state of near-panic or rage. Others were brief and poetic:

> I'm outside smoking a cigarette and feel okay, but I know it won't last (the cigarette or the feeling).

Once, she sent a meme of a baby flying through the air while a horrified woman reaches out for it, bearing the caption, "Why Mother? Why have you forsaken me?"

"I really feel for this tossed out baby lol," the email subject read.

In session, a torrent of dissociated experiences beginning from the earliest years of Ana's life seemed to force themselves into her conscious view. She expressed feeling flooded with emotion and memory during this time, overwhelmed and helpless to stem the tide. The recollection of painful experiences forced Ana to reevaluate basic ideas she'd long held about herself. She'd always contended, for instance, that drugs and alcohol didn't affect her like other people. Suddenly it became evident to her that this was not so—she was just so used to being disconnected from her body that it was hard to tell the difference between sobriety and intoxication. A similar, even more disturbing awareness developed around Ana's relationship with sex. She had, in the preceding six months, attempted to frame her rape as a singular, life-altering trauma. Her memories now refuted this tenfold. Tom had not been the start of her troubles—he wasn't even her first sexual abuser, a fact that Ana had not exactly forgotten, but had managed to push out of consciousness for years in an effort to maintain her fragile hold on survival.

Although in recent months Ana had come to rely on the binary of good and evil, there now was simply too much material for that binary to contain. Ana was not an innocent waif who'd fallen into an evil man's clutches—she was a complicated person with decades

of abuse, trauma, impulsive decisions, attempts at growth and stability, and more behind her.

"I couldn't sleep last night, I was crying and crying," she reported
one day. She looked exhausted. "Then, I heard someone scream. I
was scared. It didn't sound like anyone or anything I knew. It took
me a minute to realize it was me."

She continued, with a quiver in her voice, "What's happening to me?"

It's not that the memories that Ana increasingly spoke of were
new to her, but she had never before organized them, seen how
one chaotic circumstance led to another. How, after running away
as a child, humiliated and ashamed, her relationship with Elaine
severed, Ana began drinking and using drugs, running with a new
crowd at school. She became sexually involved with an older boy
who would force her to do things she didn't want or understand or
feel permitted to refuse. This lay the groundwork for the episode a
year or so later that she had described to me, out of context, in our
second session, when she attacked a police officer and threatened
to kill herself. The ensuing hospitalization, in turn, prompted her
parents to send Ana to a cult-like boarding school for the next two
years, where consistent ridicule and shaming were considered part
of her rehabilitation.

"The message was: You're a bad person, that's why you're here,"
she said. "There were these sessions where one of us would sit in
the middle of a large circle and the one in the middle had to confess
all the things they had done and beg for forgiveness. And we'd go
along with it and everything else because we were rated on a points
system, and you needed points to get certain perks, like phone calls
or chaperoned visits into town. We were completely cut off from
the outside world. If you ever tried to justify something you'd done
in the past, you lost points. If you said you missed your old friends,
you lost points. If you didn't finish a meal, you lost points. One time,
I googled something about New York, because I was fascinated by
the city and wanted to visit one day, and of course they monitored

all our computer use, and they said researching another city counted as 'escape planning' and took away all my points."

Upon returning home for her first winter break, Ana discovered that her parents, at the express instruction of the school's administrators, had thrown out all her belongings, the evidence of her "old self": her clothes, her CDs, her journals. A literal manifestation of history denied.

Questions of why Ana felt so unwell shifted to questions of why she didn't feel even worse. Given all this, how was she even still alive?

Even her survival had not always been a given. Endangering herself had long been one of Ana's modes of self-expression and coping, either through overt suicidal behavior or, more indirectly, by placing herself in harm's way. It was difficult for me, at first, to recognize that Ana's provocations—which often took the form of threats against herself or me—were not literal. They represented her best effort to put into words fractured experiences that had never been given a voice.

"I dreamt I stabbed you last night," she might say, then look at me askance. A part of her was testing me: how would I react? Another part was trying to communicate, to give words to an *unknown* that tantalized and frightened her, something unthinkable that she didn't know what to do with, so she gave it to me. The British psychoanalyst Wilfred Bion once described this process from the unknown's point of view. "I am thought searching for a thinker to give birth to me," he wrote. "I will destroy the thinker when I find him."[1]

My job was to hold on. To resist destruction. One day Ana gazed out my office window, the same one that had carried her into the clouds with me, off-world. She seemed absent, but behind that absence I had come to recognize an unnamable rage. "I want to jump out of this window right now," she said in a low voice.

This was the kind of moment that could understandably send a therapist into crisis management mode, where they start forming a safety plan to make sure the patient resists suicidal urges, or even consider sending the patient to a psychiatric emergency room for evaluation. But doing so would also be a precise reenactment of how people had misunderstood and mistreated Ana countless times in the past, assuming that what she was saying was what she literally meant, rather than considering that what she was saying was simply the only thing she could think of to say.

"You know, Ana," I ventured, "you don't have to threaten suicide to convince me to care about you."

Ana did not shift her gaze from the window, but I could see a mist fill her eyes and she began to mutter, "Fuck, fuck, fuck, fuck," under her breath. Then she looked at me and nodded.

Psychological growth, in or out of therapy, requires both experience and reflection upon that experience. You live, then you try to understand what you lived through. It was only weeks later when, in a different state looking back on the previous one, Ana could explain that "Fuck, fuck, fuck," followed by a nod, represented the waging of an inner war. "Fuck," a part of her felt, "this asshole refuses to be provoked, to freak out, to say he's had enough and I'm too much, to fulfill my expectation that everyone, eventually, will succumb to this." The nod was because, in my refusing to take Ana's words about jumping out the window literally, she felt that I had actually understood them.

Ana's ability to reflect on experience in this way grew, astonishingly so. It was as though she'd been waiting for permission. She became able to symbolize the raw material of her inner world through language we could both understand, rather than through threats or wordless actions. The Peanut M&M's appeared less and less. She spoke, instead, of their meaning.

"I felt like my insides were rotten. For a while I felt it literally, because I thought I was dead. So the idea was to fill myself with sweetness . . . not that this was conscious. And I needed them here especially, where so much of the rottenness would come up. Sometimes the pure feeling of it all would make me nauseous and want to gag. I worried I was actually going to vomit all over your couch. Ha ha, what would you have done? But I guess I know, really, because I emotionally throw up on you all the time, and it seems like you're okay."

Even as Ana's capacity to reflect blossomed in our four weekly hours together, her life outside lagged appreciably behind. She still struggled with alcohol and Adderall abuse. She often experienced brief, bizarre disconnections from reality, and struggled to find names to describe them. "I was sitting up in bed and suddenly I got the feeling that the pores in my arms were getting bigger and bigger. I had to close my eyes for a long time until the feeling passed. According to Google it's called trypophobia, a fear of holes."

Interpersonal conflicts were frequent in Ana's life: there was a revolving door of new friends who held great promise and old ones who turned out to be nightmares; relationships with men remained fraught, and she still often referred to her body as though it were a doll for someone else's use. Despite struggling to make ends meet while collecting unemployment benefits, she went through the costly process of moving apartments multiple times in a manner of months because of fights with roommates that, as she described them to me, slid fluidly from the pragmatic ("They said I'm too messy, and yes, it's true, my room is a crazy hoarder's nest because I'm so fucking depressed . . .") to the political ("I refuse to listen to them espousing their fashionable Marxist ideologies while telling me that they won't help cover the hundred dollars I'm short on rent").

Ana also kept finding herself at bars and shows where Tom would appear, as though conjured (what did Freud say about coincidence?), leading to a series of tense altercations that resulted in them taking out restraining orders against one another. It was my assessment, based on the information I had, that Tom had in every instance provoked Ana, but in the end it was Ana who would invariably make the first visible move toward verbal or physical aggression, and thus she would leave the situation feeling even more like the world saw her as a hysterical woman not to be sympathized with or believed.

I worried, at times, about Ana's safety and spoke openly with her about my concerns. But the lag between her progress inside and outside our sessions did not alarm me. You can't change everywhere at once; her locus of change, for the time being, was in our sessions. What she experienced and reflected on in our relationship would eventually radiate out and stabilize other areas of her life. We just had to hold on.

It was a Thursday in late April and I had a plan. My wife was due to give birth to our first child in July. Starting Monday, the first week of May, I was going to let all of my patients know that in a couple of months I would be taking three weeks of paternity leave. This would allow plenty of opportunity for the separation to be discussed before it happened. I wanted to be upfront and respect my patients' right to know, in advance, of something that would temporarily disrupt our work. I ran the idea by colleagues who'd had children while working in private practice. Everyone agreed: it was a good plan.

Then, in our Thursday session, Ana looked up at me and, seemingly apropos of nothing, said, "Are you having a baby?"

We had been working together for nearly one year. I felt I knew Ana quite well; I knew she was capable of remarkable insight. But this question left me speechless. I think I said, "What?"

She continued, "I had a dream you were having a child. Is it true?"

I didn't believe in prophetic dreams. Then again, did I have a better way to understand what was happening in front of me? I pored through the Rolodex of my intellectual knowledge. Jung's concept of synchronicity. Bion's concept of unconscious communication. My incessant need to explain, to have a theory. To give everything a name.

What difference did it make now? I didn't think I'd done anything to betray the news, but maybe I had. Maybe I was imperceptibly on edge, or distracted; maybe I'd made allusions to the future, or to notions of family or childbirth, that were just slightly different from how I typically spoke. Maybe Ana's lifetime of learning to read other people in order to keep herself safe, or her particular attachment to me, made her attuned to a missive I hadn't been aware I was sending.

"I don't know what to say," I told her. "I *am* having a child. I was planning to tell you next week."

I could see the cloud descend over Ana's face. But I was too astonished that this conversation was even happening to appreciate how dire it was rapidly becoming to her.

"You lied to me," she said.

"No, I didn't," I said, defensive. "I was going to tell you—"

"You said I could trust you. You said you weren't going to disappear. You lied."

The fear of abandonment is, really, the fear of being forgotten. Of no longer existing in the mind of others and therefore no longer existing at all. What to me was the finite separation of paternity leave felt to Ana like an existential threat, and the awareness of her dependence on me evoked in her a deep resentment.

"You might never come back."

"Of course I will. I will. It's just a temporary leave. Three weeks. It will start and it will end." But nothing ever just ends.

"You don't know that," she said. "You don't know what it will feel like to hold a baby. *Your* baby. It might change everything."

"But that's always true, to some extent. We don't know what's going to happen. I can't guarantee the future to you or anyone else. But this isn't a lie, or a trick. I have no *intention*—"

"Even if you do come back, it won't be the same," Ana said, cutting me off with an intensity I hadn't seen before. This was not the fiery combustion I'd witnessed in Ana countless times, when I could feel the heat coming off her anger; it wasn't the numb dissociation, either, when she seemed a million miles from the present moment. She was looking at me; she was here. Her voice felt cold and sharp.

"What do you mean?" I asked.

"I mean that you'll be back *with a child*. Something you'll love more than *anyone*."

Her words came at me so fast, I didn't have time to process. How could I? We cannot experience and reflect at the same time. Here was Ana's horror of a prophecy come true, the blurring of separation and abandonment, the fact that I had unwittingly destroyed her fantasy of being the one I loved most of all.

"I hope it looks like a monkey when it comes out," she said as she walked out the door.

The following Thursday, I boarded a commuter train to go home. In anticipation of our child my wife and I had recently moved out of the city to a nearby suburb, and my commute now consisted of a scenic ride up the Hudson River. I sat in a window seat next to an older man reading a newspaper, enveloped in his beige trench coat. I scrolled absentmindedly through my phone.

Ana had not shown up for any of her sessions since the previous Thursday, and had not responded to attempts to reach her by email or phone. If I'd taken the time to reflect, I might have recognized that I wasn't feeling well. I was anxious, I was tired. And I was very upset with Ana. Was she ever coming back? Was this how our story ended? An uneasiness drifted through me. Without realizing, I found that I had typed the word "trypophobia" into Google. My finger hovered over the search button.

The first time I'd heard the term was when Ana used it a few weeks earlier, and I hadn't thought about it since. Perhaps I'd avoided thinking about it.

I will destroy the thinker when I find him.

I pressed the button.

A picture of something came up. I'm not sure what it was—an extreme close-up of a flower, maybe, or a skin cell. Something natural portrayed in an unnatural way. Something creepy. Something with a lot of holes.

I turned off my phone, but it was too late. My body was fizzing with an uncontrollable energy. I felt hot and dizzy. *I'm going to throw up*, I thought. *I should lie down.* I almost did, until I remembered that I was on a train and if I lay down I would be putting my head into the lap of the stranger sitting next to me.

I turned my head and was horrified by what I saw. The older man had receded completely into his coat, so that only two beady eyes peered out at me from the shadows.

"It needs to get out," he said in a strange, slow voice.

I closed my eyes. I knew that if I looked down at the skin on the backs of my hands, I would see that it was filled with holes.

I took a deep breath and something kicked in. An engine, a reflex honed over a lifetime of relative stability, grounding me in objective reality and reconstituting the internal structures that had temporarily dissolved.

I opened my eyes just as the man beside me was asking, "Are you all right?" His voice sounded normal. His face was visible, eyes full and tinged with concern. It occurred to me that he hadn't said, "It needs to get out," but rather, "Do you need to get out?" when he saw me looking at him as though I were desperate to flee. To escape myself.

"I'm fine," I said. "Thank you. Just a little nauseous." I braced myself and looked down at my hands. The skin was beading sweat, but intact.

For a while I looked out the window at the passing scenery and focused on staying calm. Then, when I finally believed I was safe (from the photo on my phone? the man sitting next me? myself?), I started to think about what had just happened.

So, here was my psychotic core. It had been some time since I'd encountered it during waking life. But there was something deeply familiar about that place I'd just visited. I recalled sitting on the carpet in the playroom of my childhood home, moving plastic dinosaurs about, my mother coming in and saying, "Do you want a snack?" Except her voice sounded filled with anger. The effect was subtle, like a filter had been placed on the audio of my mind; I felt hot and it was difficult to move. Before I could answer her the doorbell rang, a neighbor dropping something off. I listened to the conversation between her and my mother. Pleasantries, jokes. Every word dripping with rage. I couldn't figure out whether the world had changed or I had. It seemed as though I had peeled back the skin of reality and discovered the seething cauldron beneath, exposed the lie of our nice little lives, exposed it the same way I felt exposed to the world with my skin full of holes.

Then the experience passed and the world sounded normal again. Or, at least, I chose to believe this version of reality was the normal one, because it was less frightening. And I was free to hold onto that belief when my mother returned to the playroom with a smile on her face and said, "Okay, kiddo, let's get you something to eat."

As the train neared my stop, the thought occurred to me: this was how Ana felt. She lacked something I had. The skill, learned through experience, to differentiate between what is real and what feels real in a moment of acute distress. To trust that, at the end of the day, she was not actually at risk of falling apart. That reality could not break and, even if it did, it would not stay broken.

I imagined sitting on her side of the office: her fingernails digging into the couch, staring at my dumbfounded face, standing up, storming out, saying she hoped my child was born ugly, at the brink of losing herself, knowing that she should slow down, that she was tired, that she was past capacity, but then she kept going, further into the hole, and the hole within the hole, and, unlike me, she was still learning how to stop.

6

CONFUSION OF THE TONGUES

1908–1933

Rachel, a wispy nineteen-year-old woman I'd seen twice-weekly for a few months, came into my office one day and handed me a letter.

"I want you to read this now," she said, sitting on the couch with legs crossed and arms folded in her lap. "I'm too embarrassed to say it out loud, but it's what I've wanted to tell you for weeks."

Up to this point, I'd worried that Rachel and I were not building a solid connection. She spoke often of how much she missed her former therapist, a warm woman who cut a sharp contrast to what Rachel called my "hyper-professionalism." Rachel had been referred by a colleague of the former therapist, both of whom worked at a clinic specializing in psychosis in teens and young adults. Since early adolescence, Rachel's primary issue had been a languishing depression, but she also dealt with social withdrawal and odd, fixed beliefs, both of which can be early signs of a disorder like schizophrenia. In particular, Rachel insisted that she had severe problems with memory, despite cognitive tests on multiple occasions demonstrating an above-average ability to recall information. After a thorough evaluation, including short-term therapy, the clinic determined that

Rachel was not suffering from a psychotic disorder. She couldn't remain a patient at the clinic and, my colleague believed, she would benefit from seeing someone familiar with the nebulous midpoint of psychological organization that we call BPD.

I opened the folded page. Over the course of three or four paragraphs, Rachel declared her burning sexual desire for me, writing that it had reached tortuous levels and now far surpassed her interest in our therapy. She described in florid detail her fantasies of our union—how she had come to understand my professional demeanor as a mask for shyness, a quality she couldn't wait to "fuck out of" me—and I read them, paper covering my flushed face, while Rachel sat a few feet away, patiently waiting for me to finish.

A hundred years earlier—or, troublingly, in the modern era with an unethical therapist*—Rachel's letter might have been interpreted as a frank proposal from one adult to another, a seduction. It was, in fact, this very phenomenon that dragged Freud back into the muck of clinical work after believing he'd left it behind. Around the same time that hysteria seemed to be disappearing into the sea of neurosis, and fantasy theory was emerging to guide the psychoanalytic treatment of neurosis, Freud was increasingly receiving the same disturbing report: male analysts were sleeping with their female patients. So alarmed was he by these accounts—and the threat he accurately saw in them to the survival of everything he had worked to create—that, in 1915, he disseminated one of his only papers that directly instructed on clinical practice.

---

*Ethical guidelines for psychologists can range from crystal clear to maddeningly arbitrary—the American Psychological Association's *Ethical Principles of Psychologists and Codes of Conduct* (2017, www.apa.org/ethics/code) state that it is never, under any circumstance, appropriate for a doctor to have sexual relations with an active patient, though it *is* deemed ethical for a sexual relationship to begin at least two years after therapy is terminated. Many therapists, including myself, believe that the "two years" clause should be revised to "never," but the APA has repeatedly failed to achieve a consensus around the issue. Perhaps relatedly, the *Ethical Principles* provide no insight as to *why* doctors and patients shouldn't have sex, or how to talk to patients about their sexual feelings for a doctor when they arise.

The analyst, Freud wrote, "must recognize that the patient's falling in love . . . is not to be attributed to the charms of his own person; so that he has no grounds for being proud of such a 'conquest.'"[1] Freud referred to the phenomenon as "transference-love," a variant of the transference in which the patient, in the regressed and vulnerable state endemic to an analytic session, unconsciously imbued the analyst with qualities of past loves, especially parental figures. He had experienced this with Ida Bauer, or at least believed he had, though Ida had never expressed her feelings so plainly as to represent a solicitation, and Freud never considered that their relationship might turn amorous. It had been intuitive to him in 1900 that an analyst held very real power over his patient; now, in 1915, he felt obliged to acknowledge this fact publicly. If the analyst couldn't find a way to get over himself, Freud wrote, he would force the patient into the "inescapable fate" of either fleeing analysis or submitting to a tryst. Wouldn't the latter be giving the patient what she wanted? No, Freud said, because it was not really you that she wanted. Sex would gratify the impulse without helping the patient to understand that impulse. Even more, it would make returning to a professional, therapeutic relationship impossible.

Neither Freud nor anyone else seemed to appreciate the irony of the situation: after psychoanalysis's abandonment of seduction theory, the hysteria patient had been restored to her designation as seductress—the siren luring sailors with her song, the witch ensnaring innocents with her spell, the difficult patient compelling physicians to administer sadistic and ineffective treatments. And Freud did not disabuse his readers of this idea. The patient *was* being seductive; it was the analyst's job to resist the seduction. He must resist it because the patient employed it either in a state of regression—unconsciously transferring old feelings onto a new relationship—or manipulation: using her love, Freud wrote, as a way to resist the challenging work of analysis.

My mind raced by the time I reached the end of Rachel's letter. I felt mortified, I felt paralyzed. I felt excited, too—the kind of excitement that borders on terror. I was well aware of Freud's theory of transference-love: as a kind of displacement, which was meant to qualify my excitement; as a kind of resistance, which was not inconsistent with Rachel's declaration that her desire for me overruled her interest in therapy. I knew from my training that this was a thing that happened and there was work to be done. But I was not in a state to think through any of it. Muscle memory took over: I folded the paper along its creases and handed it back to Rachel.

Immediately, to my great shock, she crumpled it into a ball and threw it on the floor. She looked down at her feet. There was a long pause. Rachel said she felt rejected.

I still felt off-balance—by the letter, of course, but even more by the uncomfortable mixture of emotion and sensation Rachel's words had evoked in me. "I want to talk about what you're feeling," I said. "But first I need to be clear with you that we cannot and will not have a sexual relationship."

I thought—to the extent that I was thinking—that reinforcing this inviolable boundary would be important if we were to safely explore Rachel's feelings for me. Her reply confused me further.

"The idea of having sex with you is horrifying," she said. "I don't want that. If anything I wanted you to assure me we wouldn't."

I had assumed Rachel felt rejected because she saw my returning the letter as the spurning of her advance. But if that were the case, and if she'd truly been hoping that I would turn her down, then shouldn't she now feel relieved? Was she only saying she wasn't interested in sex to save face? And why was the woman in front of me, her eyes downcast on her shuffling feet, calling to mind a child being scolded more than the bold seductress whose letter I'd just read? I had reached the end of the rope tossed out by Freud in 1915. He had prepared me for such an encounter, but he couldn't explain it to me.

Rachel looked up at me. "I worked really hard on that letter."

It occurred to me that there was another meaning to Rachel writing her thoughts down, apart from her being embarrassed to speak them. She had given me something that she'd *made*. A product of her creativity. The salacious content—the seduction—had absorbed my attention, but to her the underlying structure was more important. She had handed me a piece of herself, and I had folded it up and handed it back without a word.

Rachel recalled a memory—given her tendency to feel like she had no memory at all, this was striking in and of itself. When she was eight years old, Rachel gave a drawing she'd made in school to her father, a disturbed man who abused her throughout childhood. He never hit her, she said, but she'd often wished he would as an alternative to the incessant debasements she had to endure. He seemed to resent her being a girl: at times, he'd call her ugly, worthless to men and thus worthless in general; at others, he accused her, a quiet girl who struggled to tolerate even the mildest social interaction with peers, of being a slut.

"Anyway," she said, "he took the picture I wanted him to see and he crumpled it into a ball, without even looking at it, and threw it on the floor."

The letter was not a proposition for sex. It was Rachel's attempt to reach me, to be seen by me, especially in a way that her father had failed to see her. He had only seen a sexual object, and through his repeated abuse Rachel came to confuse love with being objectified. She offered me seduction because she felt *something* for me—a nascent connection I had worried wasn't there—and assumed that her sexuality was the only part of her that I, or anyone, might value. How many men before me had taken her self-objectification at face value, pursuing Rachel as a sexual "conquest" without a second thought, overlooking signs of her vulnerability and discomfort under the justification that they were giving her what she wanted? I, too, had briefly confused Rachel's wish to be understood with lust.

We arrived at a place of greater understanding partly thanks to Freud: he advocated above all else that analysts delay the gratification of impulse in order to grant insight the time it needs to seep into our consciousness. Freud's guidance was necessary but insufficient:

as with Ida Bauer, he would have given too little weight to Rachel's lived experience, and when that experience altered the course of his universal theory, he would have accused her of resisting the truth. Fortunately, his had not been the only voice in my head.

Sándor Ferenczi was the kind of genius history tends to forget. His compassion for human suffering was destined to flail in the rapid current of Freud's psychoanalysis or any mainstream cultural movement. Unlike Freud, Ferenczi championed social reform, advocating for the legalization of homosexuality and the civil rights of sex workers—both marginalized groups in turn-of-the-century Europe and ones that Freud's psychoanalysis would eventually regard as suffering from mental illness. Unlike Freud, also, Ferenczi never lost his focus on clinical work, prioritizing helping patients over reifying theory. Most of all, Ferenczi saw and presented himself as fallible. Earlier in his career Freud had been a reflective young man, open to doubt and ambiguity, but in the years following the publication of the dream book he became less and less interested in checking his assumptions. Ferenczi, on the other hand, never stopped questioning who he was, what he believed, and why. He was the shadow-Freud, unwitting progenitor of the underground path of BPD to which hysteria was relegated.[2]

A small, pensive Hungarian-born Jew, Ferenczi's early professional trajectory was similar to Freud's. Although they would not meet until 1908, both studied medicine at the University of Vienna—though Ferenczi would ultimately spend most of his career in his home city of Budapest—and both were drawn in the 1890s to hysteria and its treatment. But at nearly every turn Ferenczi was insecure where Freud was confident, overexcited where Freud was restrained, idealistic where Freud was pragmatic. As a result, the shadow-Freud spent his life and career, fittingly, in Freud's shadow.

This fate was sealed because, despite Ferenczi's vision as a theorist and compassion as a clinician, he adhered to Freud with a childlike devotion. After their first meeting in 1908, they were inseparable for the next decade and very close for the one after that. For a while their relationship, if imbalanced in power, served them both. Ferenczi's keen eye and willingness to question everything—even himself, unceasingly—produced new and often shocking ideas that Freud could then synthesize into his mainstream corpus. It was, in fact, Ferenczi's observations of the analyst-patient relationship that established transference as a pillar of psychoanalytic theory and practice. In exchange for such insights, Freud provided the paternal validation Ferenczi had craved since childhood, when his father died and left him to struggle along with eleven brothers for the attention of a strict and emotionally detached mother.[3]

But this exchange, uneven from the start, teetered on a razor's edge as the psychoanalytic movement expanded over the first two decades of the twentieth century. Ferenczi increasingly lived in fear of displeasing Freud, and Freud made a sport out of being displeased. Once, Ferenczi misunderstood Freud's instructions on how to reply to a letter, causing Freud to accuse him of "false obedience."[4] Rather than defend his actions as a genuine mistake, Ferenczi descended into one of several self-analyses in which he sought to retroactively validate Freud's claim—to uncover how and why he had unconsciously undermined the man whom he had begun to refer to simply as "the Professor."

If Freud was waging an inner war between his own radical and conservative tendencies, Ferenczi endured an internal cold war between his desire for dependence on the man who fluctuated in his eyes between father and deity, and his competing desire for independence. Every aspect of Ferenczi's life became enmeshed with Freud's, including his love life, which produced one of the strangest chapters of psychoanalytic history: the blurred treatment-romance between Ferenczi and his shadow—Ida Bauer, a young woman named Elma Palos.

In 1900, a twenty-seven-year-old Ferenczi began an affair with Gizella Palos, an intelligent, unhappily married woman who he'd known since childhood. Never one for firm boundaries, as we will see, Ferenczi could not help but relate his intense love affair to the intensity of psychoanalytic work, and in 1909 he wrote to Freud about Gizella as though seeking supervisory advice for a patient. Specifically, Ferenczi described a conversation he'd had with Gizella about the complicated transference informing their relationship—not from "patient" to "analyst," but of *his* transference to *her*. "Evidently I have too much in her," he wrote, followed by a list of roles in which he'd unconsciously cast Gizella: "lover, friend, mother, and, in scientific matters, a pupil—that is to say, a child."[5]

Though Ferenczi had been a primary author of the transference concept, Freud was disturbed to see his Hungarian friend apply it to himself in this way. The idea that an analyst could learn more about himself through working with a patient—which Ferenczi called "mutual analysis"—flew in the face of Freud's contention that analysts should already know themselves completely by going through the analysis required for them to enter the profession. Ferenczi seemed to be suggesting that there were, in fact, two people in the room! Not an object (the all-knowing analyst) and a subject (the ill patient), but two subjectivities trying to understand one another.

In his reply to Ferenczi's letter, Freud asked pointedly whether trying to psychoanalyze the relationship with Gizella might "sin against the intentions of love." In other words, would Ferenczi kindly keep psychoanalysis out of his messy personal life?

But Freud fundamentally misunderstood Ferenczi's situation. Freud's courtship of his wife Martha had been, by all accounts, uncomplicated. They loved each other, they'd both wanted children, they shared a traditional vision of gender roles and family dynamics. Ferenczi was, on each of these points, utterly ambivalent. He loved Gizella, yet for years dissuaded her from divorcing her husband. He said he wanted children yet remained involved with this married woman who, in 1909, was in her mid-forties. And he harbored secret fantasies of Elma, Gizella's then twenty-one-year-old elder daughter.

In 1911, despite Freud's caution to keep love and work separate, Ferenczi sent Elma to see Freud for analysis, after Gizella expressed concern over her daughter's stormy disposition and chaotic romantic life. Freud quickly concluded that Elma suffered from mild schizophrenia,* again placing the situation outside his domain, this time by giving her a diagnosis deemed untreatable by psychoanalysis. Undeterred, Ferenczi began treating Elma himself about six months later. Freud could scarcely contain his disapproval: "I fear that it will go well up to a certain point and then not at all," he wrote to his friend.[6]

Not long after, Elma's lover at the time shot himself in a gesture of romantic violence. She appeared at her next session with Ferenczi in abject despair, and Ferenczi felt beset by feelings of rage and a desire to protect Elma. His own reaction surprised him and, as he reported to Freud, rattled his usual efforts to maintain a "cool detachment" with patients. Ferenczi did not share the extent of his deviation—it is documented only decades later, in a 1966 letter from Elma to Michael Balint, one of Ferenczi's most influential protégés. "Sándor got up from his chair behind me, sat on the sofa next to me and, considerably moved, kissed me all over and passionately told me how much he loved me and asked if I could love him too," she wrote. "Whether or not it was true I cannot tell, but I answered 'yes' and—I hope—I believed so."[7]

Freud's 1915 paper on transference-love was years away, and Ferenczi did not pause long enough to consider either the meaning behind his behavior or the harm it would cause. Instead he leaned into his impulses, rationalizing them as validation of a long-standing fantasy. Elma, he concluded, could give him everything he wanted, even the child that her mother's body could no longer produce. The

---

*Throughout this book I use the term "schizophrenia" to refer to a spectrum of psychotic disorders that have gone by many names over the course of history and have often been as misunderstood as BPD. Even when historical figures used the term, as Freud did here, it must be seen as existing in its historical context and not necessarily comparable to how mental health professionals would understand it today.

extent of Ferenczi's inclination to dissolve boundaries finally dawned on the Professor: Freud instructed his friend to break off treatment with Elma, to stay with him in Vienna, and, above all, "don't decide anything yet."[8]

But it was too late. Freud knew Ferenczi was committing a grave error in judgment, but he lacked the clinical prowess to help him. In a letter to Gizella, Freud hypothesized that Ferenczi was acting out a displaced rage he felt toward his mother which, once resolved, would set him on the proper course of reuniting with Gizella. But Freud's unidirectional psychology, which only allowed one person to have thoughts and feelings at a time, could not account for what Gizella did next: consent to her longtime lover's cruel and bizarre request to marry her daughter. Freud could not comprehend the collective madness brewing in this rat's nest of emotionally damaged people, the collusion and complicity into which he, too, was being pulled.

"Marriage with Elma seems to be decided," Ferenczi wrote to Freud in December 1911. "What is still missing is the fatherly blessing."[9] Freud gave it, on one condition: before the marriage took place, Freud and Ferenczi must both analyze Elma in order to resolve her psychological problems, affirming her role as the sick patient and the two analysts as the healthy doctors. What ensued was a waking nightmare, a *folie à trois*, untenable and destined to crumble under reality's weight. Throughout the spring of 1912, Elma bounced between Vienna and Budapest in disorienting, overlapping analyses with Freud and Ferenczi intended to render her psychologically healthy enough to marry Ferenczi. Freud's compartmentalization had thoroughly dissolved, as had Ferenczi's compassion. Elma grew increasingly despondent and mute; Gizella's usual vivacity, meanwhile, eroded into a resigned depression.

By August, Ferenczi finally understood that both women were being tortured and that the marriage proposal was a fantasy of his, made monstrous by his efforts to realize it. He cut off ties with Elma, personal and professional—not that there was any longer a distinction between the two. By this point an abrupt end was probably the only plausible course of action, though it also served to pour salt on a festering wound: after months of dizzying interrogation, Elma was abandoned.

'   "I told you how terribly impatient I am, how I burn with desire," Elma wrote to Ferenczi in a state of desperate confusion. "It is a very, very good thing for me to be with you; I don't think there could be anything better. . . . I also feel really a little like your child, so much do I wish to be led by you. Only if we had our child could I feel as if I were your wife. . . . Write to me once, one single time, honestly, the way one speaks to an adult, and tell me what you really feel!"[10]

Though Ferenczi would not fully appreciate for another two decades what had transpired or his role in it, the ordeal left him wracked with pain. This was evident in references to his guilty feelings in letters and diary entries over proceeding years, and even more in the fact that Ferenczi never published a word about Elma. Freud had been eager to write about his treatment of Ida Bauer, and, once he'd established in his own mind that he and psychoanalysis held no liability for the treatment's failure, eager to share his account with the world. Ferenczi never felt so assured. He resumed an ambivalent relationship with Gizella, who left her husband in 1917. Under continued pressure from the Professor, Ferenczi married her in 1919.

Only Freud seemed to emerge from the episode unscathed, even satisfied. The girl he'd deemed unanalyzable had, in the end, not benefited from analysis. Ferenczi had overcome his Oedipal conflicts by marrying "the woman he loved," as Freud would later write.[11] Perhaps most importantly, the whole affair served to validate Freud's belief that psychoanalysis required an analyst to be free of even the trace of illness, while a patient must be rife with it. "Mutual analysis is nonsense,"[12] Ferenczi wrote to Freud in a letter filled with self-loathing, shortly after ending the relationship with Elma. Freud accepted his friend's supplication with the benevolence of a dictator.

Elma fled to the United States and married an American sailor, the final link in her chain of tumultuous, unhappy relationships. She returned to Europe periodically to visit her mother and Ferenczi, now her stepfather, who acted gently toward her but never made amends in the way that would have mattered: by explaining what had happened and why. As a result, Elma held fast to a singular, unrevised self-narrative, the one she'd been compelled to adopt during a time of shared delusion perpetuated by two confused men and her dissociated mother: the story of the child-seductress, who had ensnared an unsuspecting victim without realizing what she was doing, believing her intentions to be honest and good when in truth they were wicked. The tenacity of this story is plainly apparent in her 1966 letter to Balint, penned when she was seventy-eight years old.

"When I first saw him again we were both somewhat embarrassed, but later on the situation became natural," she wrote. "My evil nature had disappeared by then."[13]

Just as mainstream psychoanalysis was moving away from its focus on female hysteria, the issue of *male* hysteria—the severed thread neglected since Prichard's "moral insanity" had fallen out of fashion at the turn of the century—suddenly reemerged, catalyzed not by the inner wars of Freud or Ferenczi but the outer one tearing through the European continent.[14]

The Great War, which began in 1914, threatened psychoanalysis in the way it threatened all aspects of life: by plunging stability into chaos, disrupting travel and communication, conscripting large portions of the male population to arms, and sending countless more into emigration and exile. But the war also posed a more particular threat to Freud's movement, in the form of a new kind of illness. As wounded soldiers returned home, veterans' hospitals were overwhelmed by cases of "war neurosis": men who'd gone to war of sound mind and returned shaken and enfeebled, suffering from nervous attacks, violent outbursts, nightmares, and physical complaints of no obvious medical origin. If psychoanalysis were to justify its ambitions for medical authority, then it would need to be able to explain what was happening to these men.

Charles Samuel Myers, a British physician and member of his country's nascent Psychological Society—psychoanalysis had not yet crossed the English Channel—referred to these veterans as suffering from "shell shock."[15] It was a rare diagnostic label in the history of medicine, directly associating an external event—the explosion of bombs—with the development of psychological symptoms. But even as the term gained purchase in popular use, it made almost no clinical impact. The Psychological Society was an academic group whose members had little interest or experience in treating emotional illness; they concluded, to Myers's frustration, that shell shock was a regrettable, incurable consequence of war. Besides, even if these leading British minds had wanted to treat the condition, they had no established psychotherapies of their own—treatment in England at the time was still under the sole purview of psychiatrists and other physicians. With regard to a talking cure, psychoanalysis stood alone.

Freud and Ferenczi, in typical fashion, were equally drawn to war neurosis but for different reasons. Freud acknowledged the traumas inherent to war—and privately wrote to Ferenczi about fearing for the lives of his sons, who were enlisted—but saw war neurosis primarily as an opportunity to expand the psychoanalytic movement. If people looked to psychoanalysis to explain war neurosis, perhaps he could redirect their attention to his broader theories of universal human experience.

"I should now like to suggest that we leave the dark and dismal topic of traumatic neurosis and study the workings of the psychic apparatus by reference to one of its earliest forms of *normal* activity," he wrote in the opening pages of his 1920 monograph, *Beyond the Pleasure Principle*.[16] It was in this work that Freud wrote most extensively about the "repetition compulsion," a major contribution to our understanding of the human unconscious, yet also one he described with a persistent bemusement. How odd, Freud said, that we are drawn to reconstruct painful memories when by all accounts a feeling organism should want to avoid them. He postulated a universal "death drive" that competed with the human drive for pleasure, an idea that even his most loyal adherents would express confusion over for decades to come. As ever, there was something useful and true in the controversial notion that we are all born with a desire to self-destruct. But did the death drive equally explain, as Freud contended, a soldier suffering from war neurosis and a child continuing to play a game that left him frustrated? It seems more likely that Freud was trying to explain the destruction ravaging Europe without yielding theoretical ground—that is, by attributing everything to innate and universal fantasy, and nothing to the impact of traumatic reality.

Ferenczi was more inclined to see war neurosis as a humanitarian crisis—unlike Freud, he observed the condition firsthand and treated those suffering from it beginning in 1916, when he became director of a veterans' ward at a hospital in Budapest. Like Myers in England, Ferenczi identified cases of war neurosis that would, during the next global war, be called "combat stress," and would today be labeled as "post-traumatic stress": men whose psyches appeared to have been shattered by the horrors witnessed on the front lines. But Ferenczi also observed men with more complicated histories; men who, more in line with the morally insane of Prichard's day or the slave-beating Cretan of Galen's, seemed to *already* have been teetering on the brink of sanity, and for whom the atrocities of battle served less as a singular trauma than a tipping point. "It turned out that the year before the shock of the war he had lost a father, two brothers (through the war), and a wife through unfaithfulness," Ferenczi wrote about a patient he interviewed in January 1916. "When such a man then has to lie for twenty-four hours underneath a corpse, it is difficult to say how much of his neurosis is due to war trauma."[17]

At first, Freud was encouraging of his Hungarian friend's work on war neurosis before turning sharply against it. He took pains to minimize the impact of Ferenczi's two published papers on the topic: the first Freud held back from any widespread channels of distribution; the second, included in a collection of papers on the subject, Freud scarcely referenced in the publication's foreword, which he knew his readers would look to for guidance in terms of which contributions to regard as most significant.

So, in the end, Freud's vision won out: male violence and its effects on men would be regarded—or, rather, would continue to be regarded—as the natural order of things. It struck a definitive blow against medicine's sporadic attempts to "ungender" hysteria. Men's erratic behavior, including their violence, would not be read as illness in the same way it was for women. But it also meant that, because men who were suffering were not seen as ill, they would be discouraged from seeking treatment. Despite possessing more sophisticated theory and technique than his British counterparts in The Psychological Society, Freud was no more successful than Myers in treating the mental wounds of men limping home from war—and seemingly less interested in doing so.

Ferenczi's interest had always been, first and foremost, in the therapeutic situation. But his attachment to Freud as "revered mentor and unattainable model," as the Hungarian wrote in a 1930 letter reflecting on the early years of their relationship, meant that even as their personal and professional differences became more apparent, Ferenczi tried desperately to remain in Freud's tent.[18] By the 1920s many of the first-generation analysts, such as Alfred Adler and Carl Jung, had given up on trying to integrate their ideas with Freud's, opting instead to leave psychoanalysis and found their own schools of thought. But Ferenczi held on, writing a monograph in 1924 with Otto Rank—whom Freud would excommunicate later that year for criticizing the primacy that psychoanalysis afforded to the Oedipus complex—in which the authors tried to espouse their allegiance to Freud while at the same time criticize the dogmatic trends they saw growing in the Professor's movement. They assailed the Jungians for forcing individual data to fit broad theories, knowing full well that Freud, probably more than Jung, suffered from the same compulsion. They challenged the idea that patients should be dismissed as unanalyzable if they demonstrated wild transferences. Ultimately, they cut to the heart of where mainstream analysis seemed to be headed, a place in which the analyst held absolute authority, immune to criticism or revision: "[Just because] Freud once uttered the sentence, 'Everything which impedes the analytic work is resistance,' one should not, every time the analysis comes to a standstill, simply say, 'this is resistance.'"[19]

In the postwar tumult, Ferenczi considered emigrating to Vienna or Berlin to join the analyst communities there. He ultimately chose to remain in Budapest, the city he loved, until his death, punctuated by visits to New York and various European cities to give lectures and meet with colleagues. Had Ferenczi relocated to live in Vienna near Freud, his shadow-path might have been consumed entirely by the Professor's illuminated one. But, with a buffer between them, Ferenczi spent more and more time with his ambivalence. He saw more clearly than ever before how he had served as an instrument in Freud's machinations, driving away friends who had shared Ferenczi's passion for treatment, like Otto Rank. Though Freud wished Ferenczi to become more involved in championing psychoanalysis, the Hungarian increasingly shied away from the spotlight, focusing instead on his clinical work. Ideas of his that had been developing for years, but had been inhibited by the Professor's looming countenance, began to take firmer shape.

Freud had been well suited to theorize on seduction: raised in an environment of sexual mischief with a thrice-married father and an affectionate, attractive mother; trained as a biologist to seek cause-and-effect relationships underlying even the most complex phenomena; keenly aware of how power dynamics determined the fate of individuals in professional and intimate settings alike. The greatest psychological wound, to Freud, was having the will of another imposed on your own: being made to do something you did not truly want to do. His shift to fantasy was, in some ways, an internalization of the original seduction dynamic: instead of illness emerging when one person dominated another, it emerged when a part of one person dominated another part of that same person.

Ferenczi experienced the world differently. Reality was not so solid for him, the line between inside and outside not so clearly cut. His mother's persecutions had made affection and criticism indistinguishable, a dynamic he recreated with Freud. While Freud published unselfconsciously of his boyhood "teacher in sexual matters," Ferenczi wrote with shame in his diary and private letters of masturbatory habits that had begun in youth, or the time the family maid "pressed [his] head between her legs."[20] When Ida Bauer left her analysis, Freud never heard from her again. But Ferenczi, until the day he died, knew details of Elma Palos's listless existence, and while he never took direct measures to rectify his treatment of her, he did something Freud had refused to do: he thought about the experience and tried to learn from it.

In 1929, as his health began to fail from the anemia that would eventually kill him, Ferenczi wrote to Freud expressing a new opinion, honed through his reflections on the past and his ceaseless work with patients—"I am, above all, an empiricist"—that psychoanalysis was systematically "overestimating the role of fantasy and underestimating that of traumatic reality."[21]

Freud responded by trying to dissuade Ferenczi from this line of thinking, going so far as to suggest his ideas might represent a kind of neurosis emerging from Ferenczi's anemia. Exasperated, Ferenczi wrote more pointedly than ever to his idol in a letter from January 1930: "I do not share your view that the therapeutic process is negligible or unimportant, and that simply because it appears less interesting to us [than broader theory] we should ignore it, too."[22] The schism grew, and by August 1932 Ferenczi had completed a major, if belated, reckoning with the man who had defined his career and, in many respects, his life. Freud "could tolerate my being a son only until the moment when I contradicted him for the first time," Ferenczi wrote in his diary.[23]

The next month, September of 1932, eight months before his death at age fifty-nine, Ferenczi presented a paper to the International Psychoanalytic Congress in Wiesbaden, Germany. In it he laid forth the revolutionary insight that could only have been arrived at through the sum total of who he was and what he had experienced, from the early chaos of childhood to the unbounded mess of his romantic entanglements to his emergence from a fog of sycophancy that had only truly dissipated over the preceding two years.

Echoing Freud's hysteria speech over three decades earlier, and presenting it to a psychoanalytic audience nearly as unsympathetic to him as the 1896 psychiatric audience had been to Freud, Ferenczi began by reiterating his newfound perspective: trauma was a part of psychological illness, and if the illness was common that meant trauma was common, too. Then Ferenczi went beyond what he had written previously to Freud. The act of seduction did not cause the wound *per se*—the event itself was not what we meant by trauma. It was the inner experience of being the target of that seduction that lay at the heart of hysteria and war neurosis, perhaps all traumatic illness, perhaps most of human suffering: *confusion*.

"A typical way in which incestuous seductions may occur is this," Ferenczi said before the crowd, trying to conceal the physical pain and weakness of his anemia that for him had become a daily struggle. "An adult and a child love each other, the child nursing the playful fantasy of taking the role of mother to the adult." But some "pathological adults," he said, presumably because of their own history of disturbance, "mistake the play of children for the desires of a sexually mature person. . . . The real rape of girls who have hardly grown out of the age of infants, similar sexual acts of mature women with boys, and also enforced homosexual acts, are more frequent occurrences than has hitherto been assumed."[24]

And what would happen next? Freud had once said that the debilitations known as hysteria were "normal and psychologically understandable" when seen in the context of the traumas that had caused them. He then abandoned this position and recast hysteria as an internal maelstrom of drives toward pleasure and taboo fantasies; he framed its male variant as an even more mysterious drive toward destruction. How else to explain the complicity of so-called trauma survivors, who reacted not by hating their abusers but hating themselves, not by fleeing the scenario but recreating it over and over again?

"One would expect the first impulse to be that of rejection, hatred, disgust and energetic refusal," Ferenczi said. "'No, no, I do not want it, it is much too violent for me, it hurts, leave me alone.' This or something similar would be the immediate reaction if not for the paralysis of enormous anxiety. These children feel physically and morally helpless, their personalities are not sufficiently consolidated in order to be able to protest, even if only in thought, for the overpowering force and authority of the adult makes them dumb and can rob them of their senses."[25]

At a certain point, Ferenczi said—and at this moment, I'd like to believe, looking out at the large crowd of psychoanalysts, many of whom were already predisposed against him, he thought of Elma—the pain becomes so overwhelming that the child abandons herself completely. In her mind she can find only confusion and so, "completely oblivious of herself, she identifies herself with the aggressor."[26] She learns to see herself through his eyes, to see the violence as love, the disgust and guilt as her own—that *she*, not him, is wretched; that she is to blame.

Freud would have blamed my patient Rachel for writing her letter to me. He would have cast her as a seductress, probably, and most certainly as someone resisting my authority. Ferenczi, at the end of his life, knew this was not only unhelpful but untrue, and he finally had the conviction to declare that when you live in an unstable world—because you are a developing child, say, or a traumatized and frightened adult—attempts to symbolize your experience through language will be disrupted by confusion. Others who you encounter later in life may perpetuate the abuse you experienced by overlooking your confusion, even seeing it as clear intention, which perpetuates the confusion further. Maybe you really do want it. Maybe you really are bad.

After Ferenczi's death in 1933, Freud embarked on an insidious campaign to discredit his friend's work and minimize its influence on psychoanalysis. He falsely suggested that their views had been perfectly aligned for decades, dissuading close reading of Ferenczi's published papers and in particular dismissing later writings as the product of the Hungarian's failing health and deteriorating thoughts. In 1957, psychoanalyst Ernest Jones would solidify this narrative in Freud's official biography, writing that Ferenczi's lethal anemia "undoubtedly exacerbated his latent psychotic trends," and dismissing his ideas about trauma and confusion as the products of a bitter and delusional man, lashing out at a mentor who had only ever loved him.[27]

Half a century later, Ferenczi's speech and the published paper he later derived from it—called, in its final form, "Confusion of the Tongues Between the Adult and the Child"—would prove to be foundational to modern trauma theory, especially his notion of "identification with the aggressor." But for now that notion, like the man who'd developed it, would be forced to walk the shadow-path. In its conspicuous absence, the transformation of hysteria to BPD commenced.

7

LOVE

Sessions, Months 10–12

Before I was born, my mother began an intensive psychoanalysis that continued for years into my childhood. She was very open with me about how important it was to her. Once, when I was about thirteen years old, she told me about the first session.

"After I talked nonstop for the whole hour he nodded and said, 'So you're looking for someone to hold your hand and tell you everything's going to be okay.' I was furious. I stormed out. But then I thought about it and realized he was right."

On more than one occasion, long before I pursued a career in psychology or even began my own therapy at age fifteen, my mother had said that this analysis "saved her life." I didn't think she meant this literally, though I couldn't say why I didn't think that.

For a couple of years in college I spent a lot of time playing at open mic nights or small gigs around Manhattan's East Village. It was a compulsive practice: I would write a new song on the guitar, trot it out in front of strangers, and then never play it again. I wrote dozens, maybe hundreds of songs in this manner. I seemed determined not to grow as a performer. I'd hammer my way through a song I had only just finished writing that day, making mistakes, forgetting words. There was something cathartic in having a captive audience to my mess.

Only a few of my friends knew I performed and only one came to see me, unbidden, with any regularity. She was encouraging and complimentary, and would keep track of the songs she liked. When I found myself on stage and unsure what to play, she'd call out a title, though often I couldn't remember how it went.

One night we left the bar where I'd finished a set to debrief at a nearby diner.

"I liked the last one," she said. "But I couldn't really hear the words. How did they go?"

"Oh God, don't make me recite my stupid lyrics like poetry," I said.

"Please."

I rolled my eyes and repeated the words of the song, a feverishly written waltz about a jester who woos a young queen and convinces her to abdicate the throne. It switched back and forth between third- and first-person narration, which I thought was interesting, not that I could say why. It ended:

> Unsure if for this queen he could provide,
> The foolish clown committed suicide.
> (I was afraid she loved me.)
> Oh, my poor Lenore! The public always wants more.

My friend dipped a french fry into a ramekin of ketchup and held it there for a long time. "Can I ask you something?"

"Okay," I said.

"Why are so many of your songs about men abandoning women?"

Ana came into the office quietly and sat down. She'd missed a full week of sessions and now appeared at her usual Monday time without ever having called or emailed. It felt like ages since we'd seen each other. How many lives had she lived since last I'd known her?

"I want to apologize," she said.

"Okay."

"For what I said the last time I was here. I feel terrible. I don't want your child to look like a monkey. You must hate me for it."

I thought about this.

"Your absence was harder for me to understand than your words," I said. "You and I can make sense of anything you say in here. If you're *here*."

"I knew you'd say something like that. It's very strange. I believed it was safe to come back, that you wouldn't yell at me or say you hate me. But I couldn't bear to see you. Maybe I don't want to be understood. I thought about how many horrible things I've said to you over the last year, the insults and threats. Then I'd come into the next session and act like it hadn't happened. More than that—I really let myself forget. Like it was a different person who had been so angry and now she was gone.

"But after our last session . . . each time I thought about coming back, I tried to forget. It didn't work. I feel awful for my behavior, but also I'm still so angry."

"It's not fair," I said.

Ana stared at me with a scrunched-up look on her face. I stared back. It was thrilling, in a way.

"Yes," she said at last. "I don't know what to do with this love that I feel. It's probably what kept me away most of all. There's a lot I haven't told you. Fantasies I've had for months, sometimes sexual but mostly what I would call romantic, like kissing or cuddling. Part of me felt like it was wrong, but I also think it's been important. I don't often have thoughts like that . . . there wasn't anyone to cast in a fantasy of tenderness before. I told myself that it was something different from sexual or romantic love. I wrote a note in my phone that our love is 'eternal.' I feel sick talking about this."

I wanted to say something normalizing, how these feelings have emerged in therapy relationships for time immemorial, but it was the same old shit I'd said before. So, I stayed quiet.

"What is it?" she asked.

"What's what?"

"This love! This fucking feeling that's ruining my life and is also the only thing that seems worth living for! Christ!" She shut her eyes tight, then opened them again. "I don't even know you."

"But you do," I said. "We've seen each other most days for nearly a year."

"That's even worse! It's cruelty. It's abuse. I love you and you'll never love me back."

Was that true?

"There are . . . ," I stammered, filling a silence in which I might have otherwise thought my thoughts, "as you said a moment ago . . . I know it's new and you're still trying to work it out . . . different kinds of love . . ." I stopped. Ana had tears in her eyes.

"I found a photo of your wife online," she said.

This struck me as unlikely, but I'd learned not to underestimate Ana's detective skills. Besides, it didn't really matter. In the past her allusions to my marriage carried the thrum of menace—now, I felt only sad.

"She looked so healthy," Ana said. "She didn't look like me at all."

Helena, my first supervisor, once told me proudly that as far as her husband knew she could be a spy, so completely did she keep him ignorant of her patients. Even after I'd graduated and opened my practice, a part of me still saw her restraint as the platonic ideal. Whenever I spoke to my wife, Dawn, about my patients, I offered only scant details, describing a moment that I found upsetting or interesting without names or broader context. She would accept these disclosures gracefully—aware, I think, of the conflict they represented for me—by listening intently and then asking no follow-up questions. Yet when it came to Ana, I volunteered more—her first name, pieces of her history, and my reactions to them.

That evening, Dawn and I took a walk through our new neighborhood. It still felt a little magical, a verdant escape from the concrete city I'd called home for nearly fifteen years. I breathed in deep, seeking the comfort I usually found during life's intermissions. We had moved to the place where we intended to raise a family, but the family had not yet arrived; we were free to wait in unhurried anticipation. A heaviness lingered in my chest.

"Ana came back today," I said.

"Oh," Dawn replied.

I described the session as I had interpreted it: Ana's deep and confusing feelings for me, her sense of rejection, and with that her sense of being hopelessly ill. I glanced at Dawn: she stared straight ahead, taking focused breaths. She was, after all, seven months pregnant and walking uphill. But it was more than that.

"How do you feel about all this?" I asked.

"What do you mean?"

"I guess, that I have these relationships. It must have been different when I was working in hospitals, seeing patients briefly. With Ana, there's this ongoing, intense thing in my life with a person who has really strong feelings about me and who you'll never know."

"I try not to think about it," Dawn said without hesitation. I waited for more but she continued staring forward—committed, it seemed, to trying not to think.

"That's it?"

At last she looked at me. "She's obviously very important to you. And I imagine that has to do with how much you're helping her. But I don't really understand it."

That night, as sleep eluded me, this exchange replayed in my mind. It occurred to me I'd started from an erroneous assumption: that, if Dawn took some issue with my work, it would be in the form of jealousy over an admirer. *How does it feel to know that I, the object of your love, am loved by another?*

But that wasn't what troubled her at all. "She's obviously very important *to you*," she'd said. Dawn had claimed not to understand, but really she understood too well that, in some way, I loved Ana.

The problem of love in psychotherapy has been debated, often with great hedging and discomfort, since the advent of psychoanalysis. In a 1901 paper, Sándor Ferenczi described love as a delusional state of mind: "The person who is in love judges his love object to possess the greatest perfection, being blinded to any real physical, spiritual or moral deficiency."[1] Eight years later he began the complicated relationship with Sigmund Freud that proved himself right. Freud agreed, in a way, at least when it came to love within analysis: all love was transference-love, a trap to be overcome.

But even as professional ethics within psychoanalysis evolved to impose stricter boundaries—namely around any kind of physical intimacy between doctor and patient—the problem wouldn't go away. Even if the doctor knew better than to act on his feelings, the feelings were there. Michael Balint, expanding on ideas from his mentor Ferenczi, said it was ridiculous to think an analyst could ever be inoculated from loving a patient.[2] Dissent grew over whether such inoculation would even be desirable—was all "analytic love" reducible to an illusion, a barrier, a resistance?

Throughout the twentieth century, euphemisms emerged to acknowledge the love that therapists feel toward patients while distinguishing it from romantic love, just as Ana had tried to do. Polish-Argentine psychoanalyst Heinrich Racker called it "frank affection," akin to a parental benevolence. German American psychoanalyst Hans Loewald referred to the "perception of essence"— glimpsing the real person beneath the defenses employed to mask one's vulnerabilities—a concept expanded later by American psychoanalysts Roy Schafer (using the impressively bland term "affection") and Irving Steingart (who coined the inscrutable "apperceptive capturing").[3] These latter three, writing between the 1960s and mid-'90s, in one way or another conceded that there was something real about the love a therapist can feel for a patient—separate from romantic love, perhaps, and certainly distinct from transference or delusion. It was the love of knowing someone, of seeing who they really are and imagining who they might become. It was the love that the therapist depended on the patient to experience: the love that comes from feeling trusted, from being let in. "It is a curious fact that unless the patient feels understood we feel we have not fully understood him," Loewald wrote.[4]

In my last year of graduate school, I had a debate of sorts with two of my fellow interns at Columbia Presbyterian Hospital about loving our patients. Valery, a passionate and contrarian Russian-Israeli, contended that no amount of theory or technique can help someone change if the therapeutic relationship is devoid of love. "The rest is bullshit," he said.

Our British colleague Georgina, usually stoic, burst out laughing. "God, that better not be true!"

"You don't love your patients?" Valery asked.

"I love my *parents*," she said. "*Most* of the time. If we had to love every patient to help them, therapy would never work."

They turned to me. I said the conversation reminded me of a current patient who despaired at his struggles to find a romantic partner. Every time he met someone, or even looked at online dating profiles, he told me that he didn't feel "the spark," which for him marked the relationship's death knell before it even began. On multiple occasions he said something to the effect of, "If there's no spark, there's no point." It annoyed me every time.

"What a lie 'the spark' is," I said to my colleagues. "I've felt the spark. I've felt it with patients! They're a stranger, mysterious and attractive and vulnerable. It's based on nothing. The spark is an illness: talking is the cure. Talking dispels the fantasy and forces you to confront the real. So, I don't see how love could be a prerequisite to therapy, Valery. Do you love so quickly?"

"I do, but that may require its own therapy. Of course, then I'd love my therapist. You didn't feel 'the spark' with Dawn?"

He had a point. The first time I saw Dawn, six years before we even started dating, I'd felt it.

"But I wouldn't call that love," I said. "It was pheromones, or who knows what. Projections informed by unconscious, unknowable factors. It drew us toward each other amidst a sea of potential partners. But we fell in love slowly."

"Ah, this is how falling works?" Valery asked.

"My point is that patients come to us for help," I said. "We don't need a spark to get started."

"It's a job," Georgina said. "You can't compare it to a romantic relationship. You're a professional, you do the work."

"But I don't agree with that, either," I said. "I *do* have strong feelings for a lot of my patients. It seems to me more a by-product of the work, if the work is meaningful. The patients I don't feel love for are probably the same ones I don't really help."

"But is that love?" Georgina asked. "Or is it self-satisfaction for a job well done, and self-defense for a job poorly done?"

I didn't know what to say to that.

"Perhaps this is just how Alex loves," Valery suggested.

"Are you all right?" Ana asked me.

"Why do you ask?"

"You were in my dream last night." I couldn't tell if she was answering the question or changing the subject. "You ran up to me on the street in this kind of manic state, a way I'd never seen you before. You shouted and danced. . . . It's weird to say out loud, but you were wearing a dress and colorful makeup."

"How were you feeling?"

"In the dream? Worried. You didn't seem okay. The last thing I remember is I put you in a cab to take you to a psych ward, and I said I'd visit. As the cab drove away you stuck your head out the window and shouted something to me but I couldn't hear."

It felt oddly exposing to have been seen in this way by Ana's unconscious mind.

"So, I was the patient, so to speak."

"Does everyone have to be divided into doctors and patients? I thought I was the one who suffered from binary thinking."

"That's fair. I'm imposing a specific role by using the word 'patient.'"

"I know what you're driving at. That's *my* role, right? And in the dream it was reversed. Except I wasn't suddenly a therapist who knew what to do. It was uncomfortable seeing you so . . . *free*. But there was also an intimacy, like you wanted me to know you more than our relationship allows in real life. I woke up with the thought, 'He's never seen me naked, so how can he know he doesn't want me?'"

"Think of what would be lost if that boundary were destroyed," I said. "Our relationship is predicated on the idea that I care about you without needing you to offer up your body as tribute."

"That's a horrible, piggish thing to say. Yes, I have internalized ideas about being a sexual object for the pleasure of men, we've established that. But I am capable of wanting physical intimacy for my own sake."

After a beat, I said, "You're right. I'm sorry. I don't mean to suggest that your feelings about me are only a reenactment of past traumas."

Ana laughed sharply, like she'd let something escape. "You're so fucking self-reflective. It can be exhausting, you know. I mean, I guess it's a good thing. It's why I know I can call you a pig, because you'll listen to me and think about it and not just get defensive. But it also makes it very hard for me to believe what you said, that this relationship is based on you caring about me."

"How so?"

"You're . . . impersonal. Unnatural. Are you reacting to me, Ana, or *the therapy situation*? Do you care about me, Ana, or *the patient*?"

"Isn't that an arbitrary split? I am, generally, a therapist who sees patients. I also, specifically, see you."

"But do *I* get to see *you*? I think a lot about the things I'll never know. Not even personal things, stuff like, how many patients do you have? How many of them are borderline? What do you really think about us? I want to know you, but also it seems that this can only exist if I don't."

"It's fraught," I agreed. "In the dream you saw me emotional, feminized. Hysterical. It was intimate and terrifying. Perhaps, in the spirit of the role reversal, that's how you imagine I see you. That I care, I worry, but also that I cannot separate your feelings from your pathology, as you cannot separate mine from my training. There's a gap between us. We cannot hear each other over the roar of the cab as it races off to the psych ward."

"In the back of my mind, I've always believed that if you knew me completely you would send me away. It may not seem like it, but I hold a lot back."

"We can never know another person completely. But I believe it's possible to know someone well enough to trust them."

Ana scrunched her face again in that inscrutable way.

"I spoke to my dad a few days ago," she said. "I mentioned to him that I was having some issues with my therapist, which was a huge mistake. When will I learn? He said I should stop going, in this businesslike way that he talks when he decides it's time for him to take charge of a situation. I got angry and said it wasn't so simple. Suddenly, I was defending you, telling him how you're a good therapist and that you've done a lot for me. I told him how you barely charge me a fee. He said, 'Why would he do that? Is he experimenting on you?'" Ana's cheeks flushed and she clenched both her hands tightly. "I know you're not. But I also don't know. I feel this urge to ask, like it's the only way to get his voice out of my head."

It had been a while since I'd thought about my fee arrangement with Ana. Had it been a decision motivated only by clinical and practical factors? Years later, when I told Ana I was planning to write this book, we recalled together her father's cynical question. Perhaps it was true that, in accommodating her financial needs, I had expected something in return. But what? An object of research that I was not yet conducting? Material for a book of which I had not yet conceived? Or was it the "perception of essence"—that I had seen something in Ana, something real, something that made me believe I could help her, and also that she could help me?

She went on. "I'm realizing more and more how I've idealized my dad. He seemed so much stronger than my mom, and he would tell me that she was a bad mother, and so I aligned myself with him. For a period in my twenties I told people my mom was dead. I thought he loved me and she didn't, because she would say terrible things. He would do terrible things but then at the end say he loved me. To my dad, love is control . . . absolute control. He used to use his body to control me, then it became his money. That's how it works with property, right? You pay for it and that gives you the right to pick up and put it where you want.

"After he remarried, he sat me down one day and said that he and my stepmom were having a baby, and that the baby would need a lot of things, which meant I would need to accept less. He said he knew my mother would complain about this because there'd be less money to go around. She and I already lived in a shithole and she worked two jobs. But he told me I was strong and would be okay, and if I was really in trouble he would help. I can see now how what he really loves is to be the savior in a crisis. That way, you always feel like you owe him something."

I paused to take this all in.

"What happened to the baby?" I asked.

Ana grew tearful. "There was a miscarriage. I've thought about this a lot the past couple of weeks. When I learned about my step-mom's pregnancy, that was right before I ran away from home. Afterward, the baby was dead."

"Did you feel like you'd killed it?"

"Yes."

"Do you still feel that way?"

"Yes and no. I hated that baby and I wanted to *be* it. When you told me about *your* baby . . . I'd thought I just wanted to be your lover, but suddenly I realized I wanted to be your daughter, too. That was the dream I'd had, you had a baby and it was me. . . . I feel sick. Like, I actually might throw up." Ana began to lie down on the couch. She shot back up, as if startled. "Who are you?" she asked. "My father? My boyfriend? My grandfather? My priest? It's too much."

"I'm your therapist."

"Well, maybe that's not enough."

What happened next was a moment of what I can only describe as "mental condensation": disparate thoughts and images coalescing in a flash. Dawn's words, Ana's fee. A lifetime of fantasies of saving or abandoning women. Wanting to be everything or nothing; to save a life, unambiguously, solely; to matter so much that, if I left, the other person would never recover. If I really loved Ana—not with the spark of fantasy, but the perception of essence—then I would have to undo what I had done, no matter how well intentioned, or even necessary, it had been at the start. I would have to give back the authority over Ana's life that she'd given me, to begin stepping down from the pedestal on which she saw me as the only person she would ever need.

"I hope you're right," I began. "Maybe that's the goal, actually. For me to not be enough for you. I've not said this before because it's only just occurring to me. Probably I should have realized it much sooner. Listen. You deserve more from the world, and have more to give it, than this relationship alone can hold."

I felt heat behind my eyes. Ana scrunched her face. I'd never felt at once so near to and far from a person.

8

IDENTITY CRISES

1939–1980

Sigmund Freud died of cancer in 1939 at the age of eighty-three. He spent the last year of his life in London, after reluctantly emigrating from Vienna to flee the Nazis. As Europe limped into a second world war barely two decades after concluding its first, the continent Freud left was transformed, and with it the illness he had sought to resolve a half-century earlier.

Hysteria, as measured by how often the term was used in professional writings and clinic records by the late 1930s, appeared to be in a sharp decline. But in fact the elusive diagnosis was undergoing yet another transition that would eventually produce BPD as we see it today, catalyzed in part by psychoanalytic ideas seeping into the zeitgeist. As Freud's psychoanalytic movement introduced the unconscious to the world, the hysteria that Sydenham and Charcot had observed—which displaced emotional pain with physical symptoms—could no longer serve as an outlet for unprocessed trauma. People knew too much. A more psychologically oriented version of hysteria would need to take its place, one centered on the subjective feeling of not having a self rather than the literal feeling of, say, not having a right arm. Freud's success had changed the very disorder he'd set out to treat.

Hysteria metamorphosed into BPD through a series of identity crises. These were crises over who lay claim to medical authority—or rather *psychiatric* authority, now that specialization had become a core aspect of medical training. Several modern scholars have now traced the path of this metamorphosis, but at the time the process was too insidious, the surrounding context too chaotic, for anyone to appreciate what was happening. We cannot experience and reflect at the same time.

The first crisis was the battle over Freud's legacy. At the time of Sigmund's death, his youngest daughter, Anna—"the most gifted and accomplished" of his children, as he once wrote—stood as the de facto heir.[1] For decades Anna had been groomed for the position in ways both explicit—Sigmund had begun inviting Anna to attend psychoanalytic lectures in her early twenties, and she started to present her own work in 1922, when she was twenty-eight—and clandestine: Sigmund secretly took on the role of his daughter's analyst over two multiyear periods between 1918 and 1929.

But as much as Sigmund had, by the end of his life, run psychoanalysis like a monarchy—conferring succession through the bloodline—he had also created an egalitarian discipline that made it impossible for any one person, even a Freud, to control it absolutely. Because new analysts entered the field by way of being analyzed themselves, analysts like Sándor Ferenczi who found their own ideas ignored could still exert indirect influence by inducting newcomers. This was how Anna Freud, loyal heir apparent of the Professor, found a serious challenger in a middle-aged, divorced, high school–educated mother of three named Melanie Klein.[2]

Klein, née Reizes, was born to a middle-class Jewish family in Vienna in 1882, and at age twenty-one married Arthur Klein, a chemical engineer and her second cousin. They settled in Budapest in 1910, at which point they had two children in tow. Melanie was generally unhappy in her marriage, and each pregnancy had brought on episodes of severe depression for which—outside of an unhelpful stay at a Swiss sanatorium in the spring of 1909—she received no treatment. But in 1914—after giving birth to a third child and, two weeks later, seeing Arthur conscripted to go fight in the Great War—she decided to give the new, increasingly popular treatment called psychoanalysis a try. She consulted with Ferenczi, the most reputable analyst living in Budapest at that time.

Analysis was, for Klein, nothing short of a revelation. At the Swiss sanatorium, her conflicted feelings about being a wife and mother had been regarded as wrinkles in a blouse, to be smoothed out through fresh air and exercise so that she might resume her womanly duties as quickly as possible. With Ferenczi these feelings were received as meaningful, her dissatisfactions suggestive of a latent desire to do more with her life. There is no record of Klein's analysis from Ferenczi's point of view, but we know that during this period he was at a particularly fertile and fraught stage of his career—cripplingly loyal to Freud yet increasingly disaffected by the mainstream psychoanalytic attitude toward treatment, and plagued by the miserable episode of "treating" Elma Palos. Ferenczi adhered to the sexism inherent in Freud's conservative streak when he pushed Klein toward analyzing children, as all women who expressed interest in psychoanalysis, even Anna Freud, were at that time urged to do. But Ferenczi was also a sensitive and compassionate listener—he realized that Klein did not only belong with children in the sense of carrying out a patriarchal gender role, but that she saw in them things that had eluded his own eye and that might, in fact, hold tremendous value.

"He drew my attention to my great gift for understanding children and my interest in them," Klein later wrote, "and he very much encouraged my idea of devoting myself to analysis."[3]

That Klein's talents were first observed in her analysis with Ferenczi is indicative of two things: one, at thirty-two years old no one had yet taken her seriously as an intellectual being; and two, her insights were in some way linked to her suffering. Having no medical degree or other credentials, Klein began her career by studying her own children—a choice of convenience, but also one stemming from the need to understand those products of her making, who sparked in her both affection and revulsion. Her three pregnancies had left her tortured three times over, and she puzzled over the patina of divine calm that the broader culture associated with motherhood. When her babies cried she saw in their faces something frighteningly recognizable, her own torment mirrored back, and at times she'd scarcely been able to bear it. Psychoanalysis offered a professional lens through which Klein could consider a deeply personal question: How was it possible to love and hate something at the same time?

Arthur returned to his family a transformed man in 1916, wounded and embittered by the war, pushing his marriage with Melanie closer to collapse. To escape an increasingly anti-Semitic Hungary, Arthur went to Sweden alone for work in 1921, while Klein moved to Berlin with the children. There she began an analysis-mentorship with Karl Abraham, a member of the original psychoanalytic cohort and friend of Ferenczi. Abraham, though less of a freethinker than her first mentor, influenced Klein in two essential ways. First, his work on treating institutionalized patients with schizophrenia informed Klein's ideas that psychotic and infantile states of mind were synonymous—that we all begin life with a psychotic core. Second, Abraham gave Klein an essential air of legitimacy, without which she likely would have struggled to penetrate the analytic establishment. He wrote effusively of her to Freud; Klein would later credit Abraham more than anyone else for her professional success. By the time it became clear that Klein's ideas were not wholly compatible with the psychoanalytic mainstream, she was already in the fold, with many ardent followers.

In the early stages of her career, Klein identified as a Freudian and tried to apply Sigmund's concepts to her observations of children, sometimes with strained results. In interpreting her son Erich's enduring fantasies of being chased by a witch from a Brothers Grimm fairy tale, Klein fell back on the familiar and uninspired Freudian interpretation that his fear of a wicked woman "clearly indicated homosexuality."[4] But she also allowed for the seeds of more nuanced ideas by listening to the patient first and developing theory second, à la Ferenczi, rather than the other way around. Klein reported Erich's concern that someone beautiful like a queen might secretly prove to be a witch, and that he even at times felt seized by a sudden fear or hatred of Klein, calling her "dirty mamma" in his head.[5] She saw that as her child moved through positive and negative feelings, he rapidly and unconsciously reorganized the world as he saw it—especially his view of his mother. Good feelings made Klein a queen, while his bad feelings were projected out and transformed her into a witch. He split her.

Splitting, that human ability to take an object like the mother and divide it into two so as to prevent the bad parts from contaminating the good, was one of Klein's most enduring contributions to psychoanalysis and to our current understanding of BPD. With her concepts of splitting, projection (the way we attribute to the object the feelings we do not want to acknowledge in ourselves), and the more mysterious notion of projective identification (the way we induce the object to *feel* that which we have projected), Klein unearthed mechanisms of human functioning that deal with powerful emotions before we are old enough to use language or reason to make sense of them.[6]

Klein's role in elucidating what would later be called the borderline experience cannot be underestimated. She laid out aspects of the human condition that had for centuries fallen between the cracks of philosophical, religious, and medical establishments. In her contemporary world of psychoanalysis, these aspects had fallen in the crack between psychosis (the solipsistic mindset of infancy) and neurosis (the stage to which a child leapt, according to Sigmund Freud, with the emergence of the Oedipal conflict, which he believed to take place around age six). Freud's fantasy theory dictated that personality development could not begin in earnest before the

Oedipal stage, when the child's world became defined by the triangle of mother, father, and self.

Klein filled in the gap: there was the line, the straight, intense line between baby and mother, an infant's first expansion beyond the singular point of the psychotic core, where the difference between self and other was still nascent. In that line between baby and mother life consists of only a single, all-consuming relationship, a relationship with the person capable of bringing you the greatest joy and most inconsolable sorrow, the person who keeps you alive and on whom you are utterly dependent. Klein's descriptions of and inferences about the infantile mind remind us today that even if someone with BPD appears trapped in an extreme, unreasonable state, it is a state that every one of us has experienced and may experience again; that we all have lived through the swirling dream-nightmare of being a person who is not fully aware of being a person, an individual who also exists in some real way only as part of a pair.

Klein's divergence from the psychoanalytic mainstream took place gradually as she continued her clinical work. She began to see children as more mentally sophisticated than the Freudians, especially Anna Freud, did, attributing wild fantasies to children and even newborns that carried the heretical implication that selfhood did not begin with Oedipal conflict. To Klein, the infant lived in a feverish world all her own, a world of desire and despair, of ecstasy, hatred, and cannibalistic impulse.

"The child expects to find within the mother (a) the father's penis, (b) excrement and (c) children, and these things it equates with edible substances," Klein wrote in the case study of a four-year-old boy, a claim emblematic of her style—confident as a researcher, fantastical as a poet—as her ideas matured throughout the 1930s.[7] By this time she had moved from Berlin to London and had divorced Arthur; a sense of creative freedom and undivided attention to psychoanalysis radiates from her writing.

The Freudians tried to debunk Klein, and some of their criticisms had merit: today we know enough about brain development to regard an infant's capacity to fantasize about tearing at his mother's breast and defecating into the wound as cognitively impossible, if we take the idea literally. But there was and is something searing and evocative in Klein's writing that drew adherents to her side against all political odds. Even her most phantasmagoric ideas were coupled with astute reports of her work with children, filled with compassion and curiosity. Hers was a voice previously unheard in psychoanalysis, or perhaps heard and then driven away: a distinctly female voice, a maternal voice, and a voice of someone who had stood, at points, on the precipice of dissolution. If Sigmund Freud belongs in the annals as one of history's great synthesizers, Klein deserves recognition as one of its great original thinkers. Her insights were more experiential than scientific, her theories disorganized and strange, yet she spoke to something missing in psychoanalysis, even if neither she nor her followers fully understood what that something was.

Klein's discordance with mainstream psychoanalysis culminated in what became known as the Controversial Discussions, a series of often vicious debates held at the British Psychoanalytic Society from 1942 to 1944. On one side was Anna Freud, representing a perspective that would become known as ego psychology. As the name suggests, Freud's school of thought was rooted in her father's late-career "tripartite model," which said the mind consisted of three structures: the id, representing unconscious, animalistic drives; the superego, representing the internalized rules of the social world; and the ego, representing the core self.[8] The ego's job was to gratify the id while simultaneously obeying the superego, all while maintaining contact with outside reality.

Treatment, from Anna Freud's perspective, focused on identifying and breaking down defense mechanisms—the ways we protect ourselves from affects and desires that threaten the tripartite balance. Focusing on defenses was the most reliable way to treat the patient's symptoms, she believed, in large part because they were the most accessible: you could see a defense at work in front of you. This approach suited ego psychology's concept of the neurotic:

someone who suffered—from chronic depression, say, or obsessional anxiety—in a rigid, consistent way. Someone who had arrived at a compromise, however problematic, and stuck with it.

I once worked with a young man in his twenties besieged by social anxiety. He avoided any large gathering, or even small gatherings where he might not know every person present. He presented as meek, impotent, and riddled with self-doubt. In one of our early sessions he sat uncomfortably across from me, clearly feeling a pressure to speak and simultaneously not knowing what he was "supposed" to say. Eventually, he said this: "I know a joke. How many therapists does it take to screw in a lightbulb? Oh my God, sorry, I already messed it up. How many therapists does it take to *change* a lightbulb? Only one, but the lightbulb has to want to change."

The ego psychologist would take this joke as a defense to be analyzed, the manifest evidence of the patient negotiating conflict between his three core internal structures. On one hand he tried to appease his superego, which perpetually instilled him with a fear of being judged by others, by presenting a genial quip that might ingratiate him to me. On the other hand, he reinforced this fear by telling the joke incorrectly and with poor timing—I did not laugh, and he would regard this as proof of his being a social failure, a validation of his superego's hypercriticism. Digging deeper, but leaving the surface within view, the ego psychologist might seek to break through the defense by showing how it betrayed the very thoughts and feelings it was supposed to ward off: the patient misspoke when he said "screw in a lightbulb"; so, did he often think, and then apologize for thinking, about the act of "screwing"? Wasn't his avoidance of social contact driven by a fear of his own sexual drives, which he had come to believe were unacceptable to others but which he also could not bring himself to "want to change"?

Though Klein had begun her career over twenty years earlier as a Freudian, by the 1940s she presented a view of psychoanalysis that diverged from ego psychology on almost every point. First off, there was no core self, at least not in the way the Freudians demanded.

From birth, she said, we were suffused with contradictory impulses populated with fantasies of the mother—the ego was less a cohesive middleman than a patchwork of the chaos from which we emerge. Defenses, she believed, were too superficial, too many layers removed from the internal world that would most benefit from analysis. Treatment therefore was about fantasy: naming the unnamed, giving language to the aspects of mental life that predated language yet continued to hold great sway over the patient's behavior and relationships. The Kleinian therapist might respond to my patient's joke by suggesting that he was trying to feed her—laughter being food for the soul, after all. He feeds despite being the one who came to treatment for sustenance; he refuses to be fed. He refuses because he knows that he will not be satisfied with the milk, he will also want to devour the breast, and then the entire body. He is so ashamed of his boundless desire that he has forsaken it, made its fulfillment impossible, in the form of social anxiety.

The two approaches were not without overlap—they were, after all, both psychoanalytic. They both treated as meaningful the speech and behavior that polite society would dismiss as trivial; they both presumed present suffering to emerge from dynamic, unconscious conflict that developed over time. The egopsychology method of interpreting defense was especially practical when dealing with someone who acted defensively—it was hard for a well-guarded patient to deflect insights if what the analyst was showing him was right there on the surface. Such a patient could easily rebuff the Kleinian's deep-fantasy interpretation—those of us rooted firmly in external reality will always have grounds to deny the irrationality of the unconscious.

But many patients were not so rigidly set in their ways: children, for one, as well as those adults who had lost their ill-fitting label of hysteria, but also did not quite resemble ego psychology's neurotic. Those patients did not present consistent defenses to be analyzed but instead would reshape themselves, like liquid poured into different molds—at one moment they might use humor to deflect, and in the next express bafflement that anyone could find anything funny, interpreting the jokes of others as literal and cruel. These patients had been shunted into the catch-all of "unanalyzable" by the Freudians, but Klein's ideas suggested a prodigal return. She and her followers forged a paradigm more friendly to the borderline by encouraging psychoanalysts to engage in direct communication with borderline experiences—that is, the points where fantasy met reality, as when I told Ana that she wished she were a wolf.

Both sides of the Controversial Discussions had vocal advocates, and Klein relied on those she had inspired to translate her florid poetry into more concrete clinical concepts, apply them to adults as well as children, and codify a school of psychoanalysis to stand beside ego psychology. W. R. D. Fairbairn was a central figure in bringing a sense of order to Klein's ideas, a banner that would become known as "object relations theory." He was most responsible for distilling her writing into a theory of "internal objects," which held that the mind is an assemblage of our internalizations of others.[9] Fairbairn suggested that beyond the drives toward pleasure and destruction outlined by Freud, there was also a social drive. We are organisms drawn to social relationships, and it is those relationships—and our interpretations of them—that make us who we are.

Fairbairn also systematized Klein's notion of splitting. He distinguished the period in which the baby believes he has two mothers—the good mother who provides the breast and the bad mother who withholds it—from the later developmental achievement when he realizes that there is only one mother. The integration of good and bad is not a wholly pleasant experience: the baby realizes that his fantasies of rage and cannibalism toward the bad mother had been directed toward the same mother who he loves so dearly, introducing guilt into his emotional repertoire for the first time. Even more, it introduces loneliness: the realization that he is not one with the "good" mother, but a distinct and complex organism among many. Wilfred Bion, who has arguably informed my approach to psychotherapy more than any other theorist, took Fairbairn's model and refigured it from a one-way developmental progression to something people are capable of moving back and forth between. Even if we outgrow the initial split of good and bad, we are always capable of returning to that and other borderline states. Our minds always add and never subtract.

Isn't this a description of those instances when Ana would declare she hated me, or loved me, and then later would come into my office sullen and ashamed, saying she felt like a different person? The object relational corpus is where one begins to find ideas that are genuinely useful to a therapist trying to help people with BPD. Michael Balint—a devoted student of Ferenczi and admirer of Klein—wrote in 1968 that some patients exhibit an "uncanny talent [that] may occasionally give the impression of, or perhaps even amount to, telepathy or clairvoyance."[10] These patients had learned to pick up on extremely subtle cues coming from other people, often unconsciously, and presumably as a way of adapting to unpredictable, volatile environments beginning in early life. When I read about this a couple years into starting my private practice, I felt for the first time assured that certain moments I'd experienced with patients had really happened: Ana's prophetic dream of my having a child, say, or the time Rachel brought me a pencil drawing she'd done in the style of Edvard Munch, intuiting quite correctly that he was my favorite painter.

Balint wrote those words in his 1968 book *The Basic Fault*, a seminal if underappreciated volume on what we now call BPD. The title referred to a type of "considerable discrepancy" that could occur during a person's development "between his bio-psychological needs and the material and psychological care, attention, and affection available during the relevant times."[11] This discrepancy resulted in a particular way of organizing, and suffering in, the world, distinct from neurosis and requiring its own methods of treatment. Klein's work had awakened in Balint and others, including D. W. Winnicott and John Bowlby—the founder of attachment theory, which would in the latter half of the twentieth century form a tenuous sort of bridge between psychoanalysis and developmental science—an interest in traumatic reality. They advocated for a reintegration of reality into psychoanalytic theory through the perspective of "developmental arrest": the idea that abuse and neglect could fundamentally alter a person's social and emotional growth, even to the point of halting it in its tracks. This helped to explain why some patients relied on splitting—associated with an early, even infantile, stage of life—well into adulthood. Perhaps their environment had prevented them from naturally outgrowing these initial methods of grappling with the pain of being human.

All of these analysts, writing primarily in Britain in the 1940–60s, were only able to make their contributions to psychological theory and our broader culture because of Melanie Klein's incredible coup. The result of the Controversial Discussions was unprecedented in psychoanalysis's half-century history: participants agreed that the field would be divided into separate schools that could stand on their own. Ego psychology, object relations theory, and the so-called independent school—which borrowed from both the Freudian and Kleinian camps, and with which Fairbairn, Balint, Winnicott, and Bowlby all eventually identified—would be given joint accommodation under the tent that Sigmund Freud had built.

Amid the background of the Second World War, psychoanalysis's crisis of inheritance thus resolved with shocking diplomacy: there would be multiple heirs to Freud's creation, each paving their own path through the human psyche and treating different manifestations of its pain. A new pluralism was promised, for mental life in general and borderline experience in particular: a chance to reshape medical authority under the leadership of two women opposed in theory but united by an interest in children, childhood, and the desire to understand and treat psychological suffering. A new pluralism for which the Freudians were, quite unwittingly, already planting the seeds of destruction, as they exported ego psychology to the United States.

———

"It is well known that a large group of patients fit frankly neither into the psychotic or into the psychoneurotic group, and that this border line group of patients is extremely difficult to handle effectively by any psychotherapeutic method."[12] These words were spoken in 1937 before the New York Psychoanalytic Society by Adolph Stern and mark the first use of the term "border line" to denote those vexing patients who did not fit into psychiatry's categories. That this tectonic shift in naming occurred in the United States from the mouth of an ego psychologist is, as ever, no coincidence.

Perhaps the most famous anecdote in the history of psychoanalysis is a comment Sigmund Freud made back in 1909 as his ship approached New York Harbor. He was heading to Clark University in Worcester, Massachusetts, flanked on either side by Sándor Ferenczi and Carl Jung, to deliver the only public lectures he would ever give on the continent. Freud leaned over the side rail to see a throng of people awaiting his arrival at the dock, cheering and waving. With an inscrutable look on his face, Freud turned to Jung and said, "Little do they realize we're bringing the plague."[13]

Freud distrusted the United States's culture of optimism and self-betterment, as well as its Puritanical roots. If Americans didn't banish psychoanalysis as an immoral Jewish doctrine, he foresaw with great prescience the risk of it being treated as a commodity. What would stop some industrious figures from doing with psychoanalysis what John D. Rockefeller had done over the previous two decades with oil: water it down to a consumer-friendly version of itself, palatable, scalable, obscured from its messy origin as a primordial soup bursting forth violently from beneath the earth?

Ernest Jones, Freud's ardent follower and future biographer, initially predicted that within five years of the Clark University lectures Freud would conquer American thought. But this prophecy would take an additional few decades, and the crucible of World War II, to be fulfilled—when, starting in the late 1930s, a wave of Jewish psychoanalytic émigrés arrived on American shores, each carrying a copy of Anna Freud's *The Ego and the Mechanisms of Defense* under his arm.

First published in German in 1936, the practical guidebook that the younger Freud had crafted was something that her father had never been able to produce amid his vast and contradictory writings. She wrote lucidly about the technique of the ego psychologist and how to catalogue and work with the myriad defense mechanisms he might encounter in patients. Much of the terminology found in Anna Freud's book remains in popular culture today: "intellectualization," "sublimation," "reaction formation," "repression," and so on, all clearly defined with accompanying case examples. "Identification with the aggressor" also appears, though in a heavily modified, normalized form, and the concept is credited to Freud's father, not Ferenczi, who had coined it in his controversial "Confusion of the Tongues" paper.[14] Notably omitted are defensive concepts that came from Klein, like "splitting."

Here was a road map of neurotic illness, embraced by analysts who had been craving such instruction for years and imported to a country whose medical establishment was grappling with a new crisis of nosology.

The war had revealed the severe limitations of American psychiatry, which was almost entirely focused on biological treatments in hospital settings. It had no outpatient branch to diagnose or treat the colossal uptick of psychological distress in the wave after wave of veterans returning home, a lesson left unlearned from the First World War. Ego psychologists were poised to fill in the gap, equipped with voluminous theories dating back to Freud's "war neurosis" and more recent innovations outlined in his daughter's book. The marriage of American psychiatry and ego psychology was swift and mutually beneficial. The former inherited a mature system for naming and treating a wide range of psychological illness, granting psychiatry purview over not just the hospital but the community. The latter was granted access to American bureaucracy: its displaced, largely

Jewish cohort was assimilated, installed into authoritative positions in medical schools, and given sway over broad policy.[15]

To address the need for diagnostic clarity, American psychiatrist and army brigadier general William Menninger led a collaboration between psychiatry and ego psychology from 1944 to 1946, culminating in a document known as *Medical 203*: the world's first diagnostic manual of mental illnesses intended for both military and civilian use, predating the World Health Organization's *International Classification of Diseases* (ICD) by two years. *Medical 203* expanded psychoanalysis's neurotic-psychotic split into five categories of disorder: acute stress reactions, the newest iteration of war neurosis, or Charles Myers's "shell shock"; psychoneurotic disorders, the "nervous" symptoms that had long been the focus of analytic treatment, including the increasingly uncommon form once known as hysteria and now dubbed "conversion," after the way psychic pain converted into bizarre physical symptoms; psychotic disorders, described as the "failure to test and evaluate correctly external reality"; intellectual disorders, presumed to stem from brain disease or congenital defect; and personality disorders.[16]

The creation of this last category represented a sea change in both psychiatry and psychoanalysis—a new focus on treating chronic problems over acute ones. Austrian analyst Wilhelm Reich had pioneered this perspective in his 1933 book *Character Analysis*, arguing that so-called unanalyzable cases did not represent a failure of the patient to properly conform to treatment, but a failure of the analyst to observe the whole person. Ironically, Reich was excommunicated from the International Psychoanalytic Association in 1934, a move orchestrated chiefly by Anna Freud after Reich began to advocate for the elimination of analytic neutrality—suggesting, for instance, that analysts try answering their patients' questions rather than interpreting questions as a form of resistance to the "basic rule" of free association. But American ego psychologists, like so many medical authority figures before them, freely cherry-picked from the work of a controversial figure, employing Reich's book during the 1930s and '40s as a pretext to expand the field's domain, which could now be said to treat not only symptoms but the entirety of personhood. The focus on personality also extended the typical duration of psychotherapy, from weeks or months in Sigmund Freud's day to years or even decades.

The American interpretation of character analysis furthered a hardening of categories between neurotic character—those who demonstrated reliable, if rigid, modes of function and dysfunction—and unanalyzable conditions, the unpredictable and inconsistent types that Reich had argued were not unanalyzable at all, if analysts themselves were willing to be less rigid. As had happened with Ferenczi, ideas of Reich's that supported the mainstream enterprise were deemed as having come from a period in which he was sane, while his more seditious ideas were said to come later, when he was insane. In 1956 Reich was imprisoned following a charge of fraud from the US Food and Drug Administration based on his work on "orgone therapy," a theory of healing through sexual energy. Pseudoscientific as this work was, Reich's punishment seemed to target what he represented over anything he had done, a shot across the bow from the American medical establishment to radicals attempting to operate outside its infrastructure. Reich died in prison a year later.[17]

By the time *Medical 203* had morphed and expanded to become the first edition of the *Diagnostic and Statistical Manual of Mental Disorders (DSM-I)* in 1952, written by a similar committee of physicians and published by the American Psychiatric Association, there was no longer a clear distinction between psychiatry and ego psychology in the United States.[18] The terms "psychiatrist" and "analyst," "psychotherapy" and "psychoanalysis," began to be used interchangeably. Psychiatrists embraced the more authoritarian aspects of Freud's conflicted corpus, bringing to fruition the old fears of Ferenczi and Otto Rank that analysts, seeing themselves as implacable, would come to believe that "everything which impedes the analytic work is resistance." Anna Freud's focus on defenses was perverted toward these ends: anything the patient did could be construed as an evasion of the analyst's omniscience—the analyst couldn't be wrong; the patient could only be in denial about his being right. Reich's contention that it was the personality more than the symptoms that required treatment provided similar justification: the analyst had authority not only to treat sickness but to shape the patient in his own image of health, which could not be separated from the act of the patient submitting to his authority.

Eventually, American psychiatry, without even bothering to create a pretext, adopted policies that went against the spirit of psychoanalysis. Psychoanalytic institutes—conceived by Sigmund Freud as egalitarian training centers where anyone willing to be analyzed could become an analyst—became elitist, hierarchical organizations that refused admittance to any candidate who did not hold a medical degree. Freud's American prophecy was realized: psychoanalysis was popular, esteemed, embedded in the fabric of society—and a grotesque chimera of its former self.

The *DSM-I* drew heavily from *Medical 203* in dividing psychological illness into five subcategories. The first, psychotic disorders, demonstrated how pervasive the influence of ego psychology had become: illnesses that inpatient psychiatrists had long deemed as biological in nature and that analysts had long deemed "unanalyzable" were now framed in the language of psychological compromise, as a "struggle for adjustment to internal and external stressors."[19] The theme of "adjustment" ran throughout the *DSM-I*: whereas Sigmund Freud's psychoanalysis had begun as a theory of *conflict* between instinctual desires and the strictures of society, ego psychology—and by extension American psychiatry—was now a doctrine of *adaptation*, measuring health by how well or poorly an individual fit into their environment. Freud's notion of "ordinary unhappiness" was replaced by a moralism that prized conformity and pathologized deviance.

Psychophysiologic disorders represented the second subclass of psychogenic illness in the *DSM-I*. Perhaps in reaction to the fact that the nineteenth-century presentation of hysteria had all but vanished, this category cast a wider net than ever before to bring into psychiatry's domain any bodily symptom that did not have an established medical basis. Conditions that would now be diagnosed as asthma, hypertension, or gastric ulcers—the biological bases of which were not well understood in 1950s America—were apt to be labeled mental illness. Psychoneurotic disorders, the third subclass, included conditions like depression and phobias and were defined as illness arising out of the variable ways that an individual had learned to defend against anxiety.

The *DSM-I*'s fourth subclass, personality disorders, was both its most consequential and most inscrutable. It described people so set in their ways, so affixed to their defensive compromises, that they lived free of visible distress—opening the field of who might be considered ill to virtually anyone. Among the three listed subtypes of personality disorders, the first was "personality pattern disturbance," defined as "cardinal personality types, which can rarely if ever be altered in their inherent structures by any form of therapy."[20] In this one fell swoop, psychiatry bestowed upon itself the authority to diagnose whom it pleased with a personality disorder, while absolving itself of the responsibility to provide effective treatment. The pattern disturbance group included, among others, the "cyclothymic personality," marked by "frequently alternating moods of elation and sadness"—a description of emotional dysregulation that would later be understood as a defining, and treatable, characteristic of BPD.[21]

The second subtype of personality disorder, "personality trait disturbances," was defined as people who disintegrated under stress. This effort to rigidly codify loosely defined personalities led to unsurprising contradiction: the manual conflated emotional volatility with psychopathy, a term typically understood as referring to a marked *lack* of emotionality; the designation of passive-aggressiveness included a caveat regarding individuals who were, sometimes, actively aggressive. The section ended on an equivocal note that would become a stalwart of the *DSM* up to its present edition: the creation of a catch-all "other" category, offered to "permit greater latitude in diagnosis" and make up for the severe rigidity of all the other diagnoses in the section.[22]

The third type of personality disorder, "sociopathic personality disturbance," explicitly assigned the "ill" label to those who did not conform to mainstream society. Here one can find the codification of "sexual deviation" as a mental disorder, which named homosexuals and rapists, among other groups, as diagnostically indistinguishable from one another.[23] Addiction also appeared as a psychiatric label for the first time in this category, branding those who struggled with substance use as immoral—a stigma that has never gone away.

Lastly, the *DSM-I* featured a fifth subclass for "transient situational personality disorders," a more formalized manifestation of shell shock or war neurosis, and the clearest antecedent to modern-day post-traumatic stress disorder.[24] Despite containing the word "personality," these conditions were defined as being brought on by acute and severe stress, such as combat—personality was relevant only insomuch as it determined the individual's "adaptive capacity" to handle that stress. The postwar era's public fervor over WWII veterans' mental health likely granted this diagnosis its own section, but it was clearly not of great interest to the *DSM-I*'s authors. They portrayed trauma as psychologically inconsequential, less a cause of pathology than a measure of how well adapted the individual already was. Eschewing any mention of treatment, the authors declared that those who were well equipped to handle stress would resolve such conditions quickly on their own. Those who did not would need to be given another diagnosis from elsewhere in the manual's pages.

Rife with holes and contradictions, the *DSM-I* was nonetheless widely adopted in America both by inpatient psychiatrists desperate for a formal system of diagnosing the institutionalized and by outpatient psychiatrists looking to expand the reach of their practice. But the manual was incompatible with the preexisting *ICD*, a system that was gaining traction among international physicians, especially in Europe. Even after the *DSM-II* attempted to reconcile this in 1968, there remained no clear global standard for classifying mental illness.

By the 1960s, despite the ascendancy of ego psychology in the US—and with it the rise in esteem of psychiatry as a field—the words of Adolph Stern, identifying a "border line group of patients" that was "extremely difficult to handle effectively by any psychotherapeutic method," rang as true as they had when spoken in 1937. A pernicious group of patients continued to stymie their doctors' efforts in terms of both diagnosis and treatment—just as hysteria patients had done to their forebears in generations past. This represented a perpetual, nagging threat to doctors' authority, which was supposed to be absolute. Stern's coining of the term "border line" had only been the latest in a litany of efforts to deal with the existence of so many people who did not fit into any known category, and it would not be the last.

Hungarian-born ego psychologist David Rapaport, in his hugely influential 1968 textbook *Diagnostic Psychological Testing*, dubbed this vexing group "preschizophrenic," though, even in the process of defining the term, Rapaport conceded its inadequacy: many of the patients he'd placed under this banner did not go on to develop schizophrenia proper.[25] Some psychiatrists adopted a term that Polish American psychoanalyst Helene Deutsch had first proffered in 1942: the "as-if personality," which focused on the eerie, dissociated nature that seemed to emanate from some patients—patients who walked around "as if" they were whole, self-aware, and invested in their lives, but upon closer analysis showed that they were not.[26] Still others in mid-twentieth-century psychiatry, though a shrinking minority, made the connection between nineteenth-century hysteria and the phenomena being described by Adolph Stern, Helene Deutsch, and others. American psychoanalyst Alan Krohn argued in 1978 that the "Victorian myths of women as weak, innocent, and intellectually inferior" that had once defined hysteria had morphed into the twentieth century's "dumb blonde" stereotype, exemplified by bombshell film star Marilyn Monroe: "This kind of woman was portrayed as unwittingly seductive, psychologically ill if not physiologically virginal, physically sexy, childish, and naïve."[27] Hysteria, Krohn wrote, had always been an expression of a woman's powerlessness in society, whether as "prey to a wandering uterus in ancient Egypt and Greece, to the power of the Devil in medieval times, [or] to physical disease during the Victorian era."[28]

Yet Krohn demurred from making his claims too broadly. He took pains to distinguish his historically grounded, chameleon-like version of hysteria from the other names and theories populating the field—the preschizophrenic, the "as if," and countless others, such as David Shapiro's "passive-impulsive character," who experienced life as a series of rash decisions made by someone else; and John Frosch's "psychotic character," an attempt to uphold the neurotic-psychotic divide while conceding the paradoxical nature of those people who were stably unstable, predictably unpredictable.[29] Even those who had adopted Stern's term—merged into the single word "borderline" by the 1950s—struggled to agree on how to apply it. Was it meant to denote a patient on the border of some other established diagnosis, a "borderline manic depression" or "borderline schizophrenia"? Or was it a condition unto itself? Robert Knight, writing in the early 1950s, stated plainly that failures to understand these patients owed to the rigidity of doctors themselves, their conviction "that neurosis is neurosis, psychosis is psychosis, and never the twain shall meet."[30]

This disjointed terminology demanded another great synthesizer, who arrived in the form of psychiatrist and psychoanalyst Otto Kernberg. Unlike many of his fellow psychoanalyst émigrés, Kernberg had come to the United States by way of South America, where he had moved from Austria in 1939 at age eleven to escape the Third Reich. Kernberg trained as a psychoanalyst at the Chilean Psychoanalytic Society in Santiago, founded in 1943 by the eclectic psychiatrist Ignacio Matte Blanco, who lived in London in the mid-1930s and was especially influenced by Anna Freud, Melanie Klein, and Wilfred Bion. This environment presented Kernberg with ego psychological and object relational perspectives free from both the politics of inheritance that had been so divisive in England and the hierarchical bureaucracy that defined American psychiatry.

When Kernberg moved to Baltimore, Maryland, in 1959 to work as a fellow at Johns Hopkins University, he was uniquely suited to bring a semblance of order to the diagnostic chaos.

Kernberg realized that no one had developed a theory that allowed the borderline patient to be herself. As she reported feeling that she did not fit in, that she was not normal, did not fully exist, psychiatry validated these feelings by casting her as a transient who couldn't settle on a way of being ill that could be found in the *DSM*. At the start of Kernberg's landmark 1975 book *Borderline Conditions and Pathological Narcissism*—a culmination of his work throughout the 1960s and early '70s, and without question the most widely read and cited psychoanalytic text on borderline phenomena—he offered a unifying concept through the revised label of "borderline personality organization." The prevailing psychoanalytic view of personality was that all people organized themselves over the course of childhood and adolescence around certain principles—around drives, around anxieties, and around the defensive compromises that negotiate between them. The borderline personality, Kernberg said, was no different. These individuals possessed "a specific, stable, pathological personality organization . . . not a transitory state fluctuating between neurosis and psychosis."[31]

All borderline cases were known to feature a diffuse sense of self. For decades, ego psychologists had stopped there—if the self could not hold itself together, the individual could not meaningfully engage in analysis and therefore must be psychotic. But Kernberg drew on his extensive knowledge of Kleinian theory to take things further: such a patient, lacking a coherent sense of herself, relied on defenses that originated from the point in her development when the self was inextricably tied to an object, namely the mother. The patient split herself and those around her; she projected her feelings out; she unconsciously constructed scenarios in which other people would feel and express the violent, churning emotions she could not tolerate in herself. Her outwardly erratic presentation—she might shift from an obsequiousness to a vicious rage; she might engage in dangerous behavior and then later express a genuine conviction that she would never do such things; she might one day claim to hate the thing that yesterday she loved—was the result of her acting in accordance with this level of organization. She *looked* unpredictable but in fact relied on a stable set of principles to process her experience and interact with the outside world, just like the rest of us.

Yet Kernberg avoided any consideration that a patient's reliance on splitting might owe to developmental arrest, instead framing borderline illness as constitutional. Borderline patients tended to have a "history of extreme frustrations and intense aggression . . . during the first few years of life," he wrote.[32] An internal, instinctual problem led the patient to unwittingly compel those around her to treat her with hostility.

His view complied with the "diathesis-stress model" that American psychiatrists had largely adopted by the 1960s, which stated that mental illness of all kinds emerged when one's genetic or temperamental makeup interacted with environmental catalysts. A version of this hypothesis exists today and has been validated by scientific research. There *does* seem to be a genetic predisposition to BPD, tantamount to a person being what we informally call "sensitive"—that is, highly attuned and reactive to external stimulation. This innate quality makes the impact of a traumatic environment worse but is not in itself pathological. The environment does the heavy lifting in promoting a borderline organization within such an individual.[33] Psychiatry in Kernberg's day took the opposite view, regarding the environment as a nudge to someone born on the edge, nature determining far more than nurture.

As a clinician, Kernberg presented himself as unfazed by borderline patients, a group long deemed unanalyzable, and he introduced several innovations to therapeutic technique. First, he advocated facing "primitive" defenses, such as splitting, head on, and to not shy away from discussing the patient's feelings about the therapy relationship. This focus on the transference would become a hallmark of Kernberg's approach. He understood that the analyst had to deal with the intensity of the borderline patient's emotions in the here and now of the therapy session; if the analyst failed to do this, forcing such a patient to reflect on her history—a mainstay in the treatment of neurosis—could prove disastrous.

Kernberg also normalized the consideration of the therapist's thoughts and feelings toward a patient, which had for decades been known as "countertransference." Ego psychologists had previously written off the concept as a blight: if the therapist experienced intense emotions during a session it was because of his being inadequately analyzed himself—a hindrance to the adoption of the analyst's necessary, "neutral" stance. Kernberg said this was not only unrealistic but antithetical to understanding and treating a patient's borderline organization: part of how these patients expressed themselves was by unconsciously recruiting others to think and feel things on their behalf.

Third, Kernberg advocated for limit-setting, such as establishing clear boundaries about when and how the patient could contact the analyst outside of scheduled sessions. At the time, this concept had little if any precedent in psychiatric or psychoanalytic theory. Patients were expected to follow the implicit social contract of patient-doctor relations—showing up at a specified time, leaving politely at the end, paying bills on time, and so on—and those who didn't were seen as difficult or resistant. Kernberg countered that some people needed help establishing that contract—they needed to gradually understand that they could feel important in the eyes of another without violating the rules that applied to everyone else.

Kernberg walked a fine line between being compassionate and observant, and displaying the authority expected of a therapist during that time—the well-analyzed doctor treating the enfeebled patient. He was disinterested in the larger social implications of borderline illness—the ways in which the patient had displaced into herself the illnesses of the individuals who had abused her, the illnesses of those systems large and small that had denied her personhood. Kernberg's sidestepping of trauma and societal dysfunction, perhaps necessary at the time for his ideas to be widely adopted, also lent his approach a paternalistic air that is evident in the few video recordings that exist of him working with patients (or actors playing patients). This paternalism would undercut the benefits of his methods in the post-psychoanalytic era soon to come.

The response to Kernberg's work—a cogent, pluralistic theory of borderline experience that did not challenge etiological norms but did introduce clear and useful treatment methods—was near-universal acclaim by mainstream psychiatry and ego psychology. As with Sigmund Freud in the 1900s, this success could be attributed in no small part to the fact that Kernberg's methods worked: therapists began to report successful treatment of previously intractable cases as a result of his approach. Even more, doctors' various disparate observations of borderline phenomena—from the more overt symptoms observed by inpatient psychiatrists to the subtle explorations of aloneness, dissociation, and the patient-therapist relationship— were at last being discussed under the single label of "borderline." Advances in the field could be disseminated easily, where previous attempts at the coherent exchange of knowledge had been akin to communicating amid the rubble of the Tower of Babel, with everyone using a different name and speaking a different language.

Borderline individuals who had been forgotten by the psycho-analytic treatment founded on their suffering, who had endured so many false hopes and abandonments, were once again receiving interest and attention from medical authorities. Although Kernberg and others continued to overlook the cultural and personal histories of such patients—severing them from the legacy of hysteria and de-nying the role of childhood trauma—they had nevertheless resolved the crisis of nosology, forging a coherent identity for a condition defined by an incoherent sense of self. The only thing that could disrupt the momentum now would be a near-total dismantling of the psychoanalytic establishment in the United States.

———

Matthew, a twenty-year-old man I'd worked with for a few months, began a session saying he was in crisis. "I think I'm a narcissist," he told me. "I'm *terrified* of it."

I asked Matthew why he thought this. He said the night before he had, after much agonizing, confronted his boyfriend Patrick about his controlling behavior: Patrick decided when they socialized and with whom; he required advance approval of any expenses related to the apartment they shared; he discouraged Matthew from engaging in any interests that did not help to "build the relationship," especially Matthew's longtime passion for oil painting.

"Then Patrick told me that, by bringing this up, *I* was trying to control *him*," Matthew said. "He said I was using guilt to manipulate him into getting what I wanted, which he said was worse than anything he had done because all of his rules were completely rational." Matthew put his head in his hands. "And I couldn't . . . I see how he flipped the conversation around on me, but I couldn't really deny that what he was saying was true . . ." He looked up at me with desperate, searching eyes. "Is it true? Am I a narcissist?"

As early as the 1960s Kernberg had bemoaned the overuse of "narcissism" in psychoanalytic and popular writing, which could sometimes refer to a general aspect of the human condition—we all have times in which we are preoccupied with our own needs and desires—and at other times described more extreme ways of being. This conflation can be traced back to Sigmund Freud, who wrote about narcissism beginning in 1914 and highlighted its universal presence in human culture: the term itself, after all, dated back thousands of years to the ancient Greek myth of a young man, Narcissus, who fell in love with his own reflection. Kernberg used the term "pathological narcissism" to distinguish the more extreme version, and his behavioral descriptions of these cases would serve as the basis for present-day narcissistic personality disorder (NPD).[34]

Kernberg saw the narcissist as very similar to the borderline: both struggled with managing powerful, negative emotions; both relied on splitting the world into good and bad. But where the borderline often cast herself as bad to preserve the goodness of others—on whom she relied for validation that she was real and alive—the narcissist organized his internal world so that he was always good, the outside world always inadequate and unappreciative. The narcissist often appeared better adapted to the world than the borderline, as he possessed a self-idealization that could be misconstrued as confidence. But beneath the brittle surface lay a tumult that, when put under pressure, could compel him into strange and harmful behavior.

As with his theory of borderline personality, Kernberg held little room for environment in his discussions of narcissism, though he did note that "cold parental figures with covert but intense aggression" were frequently found in the history of adult patients suffering from pathological narcissism.[35] In this area Kernberg found a serious critic in Heinz Kohut, a fellow Austrian-born analyst who promoted a theory of developmental arrest. According to Kohut, we all proceed through "normal" narcissistic phases, particularly in adolescence, but some of us get stuck in them due to traumatic or otherwise impoverished environments.[36]

In many ways Kernberg and Kohut were saying the same things with different language, and with different political agendas—the former working to change American psychiatry from within and the latter a vocal critic of it, calling for a revolution from without. A major difference between them pertained to treatment. Kernberg saw narcissism as a defense hiding the borderline organization beneath—the patient's tendencies toward self-aggrandizement and debasement of others therefore needed to be breached so that his underlying structures could be exposed. Kohut took an opposite approach: because he saw the pathology in terms of arrest, he advocated for the therapist to take on the role of a warm, supportive parent, encouraging the patient in effect to resume his development and naturally grow out of his narcissistic mire. Many therapists, including myself, would come to adopt a hybrid of these viewpoints: sometimes you need to challenge the patient and sometimes you need to hold him.

Kohut saw narcissistic patients as having a more fully developed sense of self than borderline patients and therefore claimed they were easier to treat, though this has never been my experience.[37] People organized around narcissistic defenses are afraid more than anything of vulnerability, of being seen as weak, which makes the therapy situation inherently unappealing to them. They are driven to point out ways that they are smarter than the therapist or already knew what the therapist is going to say. Borderline patients, on the other hand, could be described as pathologically vulnerable, porous to the point of diffusion, and their reliance on others for cohesion means that they are excellent candidates for a relationship-based treatment like psychotherapy.

I treat pathological narcissism in my practice, though most often I encounter it as with Matthew: listening to a borderline patient talk about a narcissistic partner, parent, or sibling. The two personality organizations tend to gravitate toward each other, a toxic magnetism. One person seeks definition, the other seeks to define; the borderline wants to love even if it hurts, the narcissist wants to wield power even over someone he loves.

Matthew and I discussed this dynamic. That night he had a long conversation with Patrick, which he relayed to me at our next session.

"I described the way we feed into each other. I ask Patrick to tell me what to do, he happily tells me, then I confuse his orders for my own thoughts. I told him that I was borderline for the first time." By the time I'd met Matthew, about three years after beginning work with Ana, my experience with BPD had grown substantially. He and I had talked about giving time to establish a solid understanding of the term. Matthew took this seriously, resisting the urge to google his diagnosis or broadcast it to the world until he was sure he was ready to do so.

"I'm still confused about what happened next," Matthew went on. "Something changed in him, like I'd made him angry. I explained a bit about the diagnosis. I said I was susceptible to him telling me what I am, like that I'm controlling or narcissistic, and also that it was related to stuff from early childhood. And he said, 'What even happened to you that's so bad?' I didn't feel comfortable talking to him about some of things we've talked about, but I also felt this pressure to explain myself. I said, 'I'm not saying I had the worst life or anything. You know my parents, they're not bad people. But there was some trauma—' and he cut me off and said, '*You* had trauma? Listen, I could teach you something about that.' It seemed like I'd really hit a nerve and I felt bad, so I asked him what he meant. And he got very serious and intense and he told me . . . I feel weird repeating it . . . he told me that when he was a baby he had been raped repeatedly by cultists as part of a satanic ritual."

Matthew hadn't known what to do. The story sounded preposterous, but he didn't want to invalidate Patrick or turn the conversation back to himself—fuel for Patrick's charge that Matthew was the true narcissist. I suggested that Patrick may have felt threatened by Matthew's borderline diagnosis: it made Matthew special in a way that Patrick could not bear. Moments like this show how narcissism is not a pleasant way of living, filled with self-love and confidence—it is a frantic struggle to always be on top, even if that means waging a contest for who is the most ill, or producing a horrible memory that is most likely false. Did Patrick believe what he had said to Matthew? In the moment he probably did. Narcissism is liquid armor: no contortion is too extreme, so long as it preserves the person's sense of invulnerability.

We might say that borderline and narcissistic adults come from similarly troubled origins but, starting in childhood, are treated differently. The one who grew up to adopt a borderline organization was called worthless; she was hit for being disobedient, perhaps, or praised for being beautiful enough to one day ensnare a rich husband. The future narcissist was perhaps called a prodigy and forced into public, competitive spaces despite expressing no inherent interest in them; he was praised as strong for his cold-heartedness, berated as weak when he cried.

I've treated borderline men and narcissistic women—individual circumstances can always overwhelm larger cultural forces. But there is a gendered split to these pathways, the same split found across so many aspects of life. In the world that Freud had changed, male hysteria had changed, too—finding new form in the pathological narcissist.

In December 1973, a thousand psychiatrists and a swarm of reporters gathered in Washington, DC, to hear a debate at the annual convention of the American Psychiatric Association, the organization that published the *DSM*. One side of the debate was represented by a group of progressive psychiatrists—spurred by conviction and a growing furor in public opinion—who argued that the *DSM* should no longer list homosexuality as a mental disorder. The opposing side was occupied by old-guard psychiatrists, including several venerated ego psychologists, who may well have believed in the *DSM*'s "sexual deviation" diagnosis but *definitely* believed that no one, least of all the public, should have a say in the language or scope of their authority.

The winds of change were apparent to all but the old guard. The debate—which would in fact result in the removal of homosexuality from future editions of the *DSM*—was a culmination of everything that had gone wrong with psychoanalysis in the US over the last thirty years. The field's countercultural roots—a treatment developed by Jews to help women by encouraging them to forsake social norms and say whatever came to mind—had gnarled into a towering overgrowth of conservatism; psychiatry's prestige had climbed so high that the field became ensconced in a cycle of maintaining the status quo. So thoroughly had the establishment felt assured of its dominance that it had allowed multiple opposing factions to develop simultaneously, who by the mid-1970s posed an existential threat: the grassroots gay rights activists, who portrayed psychiatry as a tool of authoritarians used to suppress civil liberty; the biological psychiatrists, once seen as the least effective branch of the field, now cutting-edge pioneers whose advances in pharmacology promised to treat even the most severe, institutionalized patients; the psychoanalytic psychiatrists, whose cries for reform from within the system had repeatedly been ignored; the psychologists and other non-MD mental health providers, long boxed out of analytic training institutes, who flocked to new, so-called humanistic therapies, such as Carl Rogers's client-centered therapy, Fritz Perls's gestalt therapy, and Heinz Kohut's self psychology. A popular anti-psychiatry movement was growing from the fertile soils of government distrust, counterculturalism (including a movement born from Wilhelm Reich's proposed "sexual revolution"), and a new American infatuation with Eastern religion and philosophy.

American psychiatry was faced with a full-blown crisis of legitimacy. And there was no better battleground in which to hash out its future than the next edition of the *DSM*. The revision that would be published in 1980 as the *DSM-III* is most sensibly viewed as a formal repudiation of ego psychology, a frantic bid to redefine American psychiatry as a discipline disinterested in talk therapy—increasingly the purview of clinical psychologists—and instead focused chiefly on biological and epidemiological research.

The revision purged all psychoanalytic language and concepts without anything to take their place. Biological psychiatry, though growing in stature, was too immature to lend a hand at diagnosis— there was still only an embryonic understanding of how brain areas and chemicals, let alone genes, related to specific mental disorders. So the *DSM-III* abandoned etiology altogether, a decision that has remained in place up to its present fifth edition. The question of where mental illness came from—whether organic, psychogenic, or a combination thereof—was rendered irrelevant to the field of psychiatry, which now centered itself instead on observable criteria through which to assign diagnoses. Instead of psychoanalytic theory, or any theory, the *DSM-III* defined diagnoses by "symptom clusters" that epidemiological studies had shown tended to go together in patients.

The consequences of the *DSM-III* were manifold. Where previously the manual had been an ancillary text for the many psychiatrists who saw little need for diagnosis, it was now foundational: psychiatry, untethered from theory, had no glue to hold itself together apart from its official compendium of disorder. It was this edition that earned the moniker of "psychiatry's bible" that is still used to describe the *DSM* today—and indeed the *DSM-III* took on the qualities of a religious text, a dogma to be followed without theoretical underpinnings. A disease was a disease because the book said it was a disease.

The *DSM-III*'s new focus on behavioral symptoms and arbitrary thresholds—a major depressive episode, for example, could be diagnosed if a patient's symptoms had persisted for fourteen, but not thirteen, days—made the manual more useful than its predecessors, in a way. Any psychiatrist could consult their copy and run through the checklists to determine a patient's diagnosis—or diagnoses. In fact, psychiatrists would *have* to consult the *DSM-III*, as psychoanalytic training was quickly dropped from medical curricula, leaving them with no viable tool apart from this new bible to conceptualize what was going on with a given patient. The manual's categorical approach to illness quickly proved to be a poor representation of real life, as most patients met criteria for multiple disorders rather than neatly slotting into one.

The *DSM-III* enjoyed skyrocketing popularity not only in the US but abroad, eclipsing all other diagnostic manuals including the *ICD*, which would in the coming years change its own classification system to align with America's. In influencing its competitors, the *DSM-III* also helped reduce psychoanalysis's stature in psychiatry throughout Europe and Latin America, where object relational and independent ideas had previously had a foothold.

In one sense, psychiatry's crisis of legitimacy resolved through progressivism: the field averted total collapse by appeasing its fiercest critics. Homosexuality was removed as a mental disorder in the *DSM-III*, scientific research was introduced as the basis for diagnostic labels, and biological treatments were framed as the future of clinical work. In another sense it resolved through desperate, reactionary tactics, as psychiatry abandoned a century of psychoanalytic knowledge in order to distance itself from ego psychology's stained reputation.

The great irony was that Kernberg's concept of the borderline personality—informed entirely by psychoanalytic principles—had gained such widespread acceptance by 1980 that it was imported into the *DSM-III* under the modified name of Borderline Personality Disorder. Finally, the diagnosis with which we are all familiar, the one I gave to Ana, Blake, Rachel, Matthew, and others, had arrived. But without context. The *DSM-III* made no mention of a continuum of neurotic, borderline, and psychotic personality organizations; nor of splitting, projective identification, or any other psychological defense; nor of any of the therapeutic innovations that had proven beneficial. The word "therapy" appeared precisely fifteen times in the *DSM-III*'s five hundred pages, none of which referred to the treatment of personality disorders. There was, of course, no mention of any relationship between early trauma and BPD, or of why the label was disproportionately applied to women. "The disorder is more commonly diagnosed in women" was all the *DSM-III* had to say on that point.[38]

The *DSM-III* defined BPD as the presence of at least five of the following symptoms in an individual: (1) impulsive behavior such as overspending, promiscuous sex, and shoplifting, (2) a pattern of unstable or volatile relationships, (3) "inappropriate" anger, (4) uncertainty with regard to identity, (5) mood instability, (6) the inability to be physically alone, (7) recurrent self-mutilating behaviors, whether accidental or deliberate, and (8) chronic feelings of emptiness or boredom.[39] No meaningful revision to these criteria has occurred in subsequent editions. BPD was here etched into psychiatry's bible, a fixture of diagnosis and soon to become a household term. But it had been severed from its history, drifting into the modern era as a name without meaning.

Histrionic personality disorder (HPD)—a term first coined by Alan Krohn in the 1970s to capture his version of the contemporary hysteric—also appeared for the first time in the *DSM-III*. I will not list out the criteria for this new diagnosis, but, suffice to say, it overlapped with BPD to a perplexing degree—perplexing, that is, to the reader who lacked the knowledge that these disorders stemmed from different psychiatrists trying to describe the same thing, knowledge that the *DSM* omitted. The section on HPD ended simply by stating, "Borderline Personality Disorder is also often present; in such cases both diagnoses should be made."[40]

Narcissistic personality disorder also first appeared in the *DSM-III*, codified as the list of symptoms familiar to most people today: unique ones like grandiosity and the tendency to exploit others, as well as ones shared with BPD and HPD, such as excessive anger and "relationships that characteristically alternate between the extremes of overidealization and devaluation."[41] Insufficient data existed in 1980 regarding the gender breakdowns within these diagnostic categories, though by the *DSM*'s fifth edition the pattern was clear: 75 percent of NPD diagnoses were given to men and, uncannily, 75 percent of BPD diagnoses were given to women.[42] No edition of the *DSM* has dared broach the idea that these conditions represented two ways a person might resolve the same core problems according to the strictures of a sexist society.

9

SELF-DISCOVERY

Sessions, Year 2

The second year of therapy with Ana felt different from the first. She would later describe it to me as the year she discovered, or perhaps rediscovered, that she was a person:

"When we first met, I became almost immediately dependent on you, in a very extreme way. It felt like seeing you proved that I was real, after going through something that I literally thought had destroyed me. Later, I still felt I needed you, but as someone who would help me, not define who I am. I started thinking for myself from the inside out, in terms of what I felt or wanted. I had always done it the other way before, from the outside looking in—what do they feel? what do they want?—or I'd just done things without really knowing why. Really, I'd spent my whole life being asked, 'Why did you do that?' Parents, teachers, friends, boyfriends. 'Why did you do that, Ana? Why?' I started to see that this was why I felt so ashamed all of the time. I had internalized what the question implied, which is that I was supposed to be in control of my impulses, that I was making the wrong choice and ought to know better."

Much of what Ana was coming to understand was invisible to me at the time. She didn't withhold information from me, at least not in the pejorative sense of "resisting" the therapy—it was more that she began to experiment with privacy. Ana had always kept journals as a young teenager, a practice she'd abandoned after her parents threw out all her belongings when they sent her away to boarding school. What was the point of recording your private thoughts and feelings if, in the end, they would not remain private, not even remain yours? Now, she began to write again.

From my side of the room, I understood that while much of what Ana and I discussed was familiar material from our first year of therapy—she continued to grapple with powerful affects, insomnia, dissociation—something had changed. I felt calmer with her, more solid, but also more separate. Intellectually, I knew that Ana had never really told me *everything* that was on her mind—that was impossible. All relationships are based on incomplete data. Yet I think that, during that first year, I'd convinced myself that I knew everything about her as a way to soothe myself, or maybe to feel important. At times Ana had surely picked up on this and confessed to me thoughts and feelings before she'd had time to consider whether she wanted to share them. Conversations in our second year often returned to this idea: Ana had the right to be quiet if she didn't want to speak, or to say no if she didn't want to do something. She worried that if she didn't tell someone *everything*—about her trauma history, her diagnosis, her intensive psychotherapy—they would know nothing, and could never understand her. But more and more, our relationship seemed to be proof that this wasn't true.

"I'm really craving Adderall," Ana told me one day. "I thought about going to find some quack doctor who would write me a prescription, but I stopped myself."

I chewed on this for a moment, wondering whether I had missed something, or if she had. "Do you mean you haven't been taking it recently?" I asked.

"Oh, yes . . . I quit two months ago."

My first reaction was one of offense. Ana's abuse of stimulants had been clear to both of us for a long time, especially its impact on her anxiety, sleep, and appetite. I'd made my concerns clear but never pressured her to stop using, and we hadn't talked about it recently. How dare she achieve an objective milestone of progress without telling me!

But wasn't that the point? For Ana to take care of herself, and to feel free to do so without my, or anyone's, permission?

"Oh, I see," I said.

"You know, I thought about dropping out of therapy a lot at the beginning, and I still do sometimes," she replied. "One of the reasons I stayed is that symptoms I didn't even know I had started to disappear. I'd bitten my nails since I was eight years old, sometimes till my fingers bled, and suddenly I stopped. It felt like magic."

This comment struck me as deeply compassionate, even if Ana was not fully conscious of why she'd said it. She was assuring me our relationship helped her even in ways we did not explicitly discuss—such as her nail biting or, now, her Adderall use.

"Not magic," I said. "I think you were so ready to get better. You just needed someone to provide space for it and, ideally, to stay out of your way."

Ana's eyes teared up. I wasn't sure how I felt about what I'd just said.

"I don't see it as magic anymore," she said. "Which is good and bad. I kind of miss when it felt like it was just you and me, and my job was to come here and try to get better. But now, like, I need an actual job. I need to get off unemployment. I've been thinking about maybe going back to school. I'm not sure if therapy can help me with those things."

"As you add more things to your life, our relationship will become a relatively smaller part of it," I said.

"I don't know why I'm crying. It feels like you're saying that you're leaving me. I know you're not. This can't be my whole life forever, and at some point maybe it becomes so small a part that it ends. Isn't that what I want?"

———

At the time I didn't make the connection, but in retrospect it's hard not to notice: as my practice grew—and became more centered on patients dealing with borderline issues—Ana began to date. We both felt the shift in our dynamic, a move toward something less enveloping. Were we seeking to fill that space, to take what we'd learned from each other and apply it to new relationships? I had been working with Rachel for some months at this point, and now began to see Blake and other BPD patients. I started to describe myself at professional events as someone who focused on BPD, and listed the diagnosis for the first time on my website as one of my "specializations," a term I'd always resisted but had been told was necessary to compete in the mental health marketplace. Even as I was discovering that being borderline was not so "special," that it was common and somehow related to the human condition, including my own, I wanted people to see me as an expert—that is, to forge my reality through the gaze of others.

Ana's foray into the dating pool was no less ambivalent. Her sexual encounters with men had reduced over the last year until they had stopped entirely. At first she experienced a sharp reversal of her previous attitude toward sex. Immediately after the rape, she had trivialized the act and demeaned her participation in it, partly as a way to reduce the horror of the violation her body had endured. Once she had slowed down enough to take an intentional break from sex, Ana suddenly found that even the idea of being touched was repulsive. She said she thought it was important to be single for a while. But this, too, was difficult to tolerate. Though Ana never specified how long "a while" was meant to be, her voice betrayed some disappointment when she told me a month or so later that she had downloaded a dating app and matched with someone. His name was Anders. In session, Ana called him Swedish Fish.

"Because he's so sweet," she explained. "Sometimes it's almost sickening. He's . . . *sugary*."

I asked in what way Anders was sweet. Ana said that at the bar where they met on their first date, they'd sat down in front of an air conditioning unit and, after a few minutes, he asked if she felt cold and would prefer to sit somewhere else. Later, he commented on how the bartender "seemed stressed" and that bartending must be a hard job. At the end of the night, he gave Ana a brief kiss and said goodbye without pressuring her to have sex.

"Is that sweetness?" I asked. "It sounds like he exhibited a basic level of respect for you and other people."

Ana burst out laughing. "That's basically what he said! I texted him the next day and said, 'I don't know if this is going to work, you're too sweet.' And he said, 'Really? I've been told I can be kind of robotic.'"

She continued to see Anders, which she found to be a confusing experience. He seemed to like her—he responded to texts quickly and at one point said, "I like you"—but he did not seem interested in merging his life with hers. "The first night I met Tom," Ana told me, "he slipped something into my drink. That's how our relationship started. I found a way to laugh about it, and I think I was drawn to how clearly he wanted to dominate me. We spent the next week barely being out of each other's sight. Swedish Fish is not like that. When I went to his apartment last night, he looked anxious and he said it was hard for him to have new people in his space. He talks about space a lot. He seems to really value *space*. Maybe he's not a Swedish Fish—maybe he's whatever they call Swedish astronauts."

After a few weeks Ana came into my office looking upset. She said that Anders had told his therapist—he was receiving cognitive-behavioral treatment for anxiety—that he had started dating a woman with BPD.

"He said that she said that he should break up with me. Who does she think she is? I hate this woman. Would you ever say anything like that? Then he asked if what I do with you is called 'DBT,' and I said no, and he said that she said that if I wasn't getting DBT I would never improve and he should *definitely* break up with me."*

"And what did Anders make of this advice?"

"He wasn't an asshole about it. He said he didn't necessarily agree with her. But then he said it stressed him out that his therapist said it, because he likes things to be very clear—that's what he likes about his therapy and that's how he deals with his anxiety: he makes sure everything is very clear. And I said, 'I am *not* clear. I am blurry as fuck.' Then we kind of laughed and things calmed down, but I don't know what to do. Can I be with someone who would listen to what his therapist said and not immediately say, 'That's bullshit and feeds into a stigma about something you don't understand'?"

"It's also something Anders doesn't understand," I said. "Unless he has some previous context for BPD, he would need time to figure this stuff out for himself."

Ana said she didn't know if she had that kind of time, or wanted to serve as someone's "mentor in the ways of the borderline." I said something to the effect of how this kind of dating—relatively slow moving, bounded, and filled with mixed emotions—was new for her, and she should take it at her own pace. Later that day she broke up with Swedish Fish.

I went to a party in my neighborhood and met a woman who was also a clinical psychologist. We exchanged some pleasantries about living in the area and our common experience of being new parents. Unprompted, she began to tell me about her specializations.

"I treat OCD using a hybrid CBT-ERP approach," she said. "And I mean real OCD, *DSM-5* OCD, not people who just think they have it because it's a popular term now."

---

*We will look closely at DBT's history, principles, and reputation in the next chapter.

"What happens to the people who just think they have OCD?" I asked.

She laughed. "I tell them they should stop taking online quizzes and refer them out." I nodded and she looked at me suspiciously. "What are *your* specializations?" she asked.

"The people you refer out," I said. I waited for her to laugh again but she didn't, so I said, "I see a lot of people who find being alive really difficult but don't know why." She continued to look at me. I interpreted her look as awaiting some context from the *DSM-5*. "A lot of BPD," I said at last, as if under duress.

She flashed a big smile and said, "Fun!"

In that moment we both understood that even though from the perspective of everyone else at the party we were aligned as two clinical psychologists, we actually had nothing to say to one another. Had this woman never woken up from a dream and wondered what it meant? And though I'd once known what "ERP" stood for, I was too embarrassed to admit that I'd forgotten. We drifted apart, each toward our respective spouses to debrief.

"How'd it go?" Dawn asked.

"If I wanted to have *fun*," I said in a harsh whisper, "I would have become a goddamn zip-line instructor. Like that guy on our honeymoon who asked us every five minutes, 'Isn't this fun?!' We all have to justify our lives to ourselves, I guess. It would be nice to understand what I do as so simple and straightforward that everyone who didn't fit the mold was just noise to be ignored. But then, of course, I'd probably get so bored that I'd kill myself."

Dawn patted me on the back. "It can be hard to make new friends," she said.

The next guy Ana dated was called Moses, which she said seemed like a bad sign.

"I probably shouldn't be with someone prophesied to lead people to the Promised Land," she said.

"It did take forty years," I offered.

Ana's premonition turned out to be right, if for profane reasons. Upon hearing of her diagnosis—a piece of information Ana still struggled to feel she had the right to withhold from nearly anyone she met—Moses reacted with a visceral intensity.

"He said, 'Oh God, you're going to split me, aren't you?' He seemed panicked, like there was nothing we could do and it was already too late."

It was unclear how Moses had arrived at this conclusion, whether he had read about BPD online, or dated other women diagnosed with BPD—or, as I suspected, had been diagnosed with it himself at some point. He himself certainly evidenced a tendency to split, and to follow his emotions in an impulsive, contradictory way, such as insisting on spending more and more time with Ana even as he said he was afraid they were going "too fast." Yet for all they had in common, Moses had somehow managed to disavow BPD, to see it as an external threat rather than a part of him. Maybe this was the difference between the borderline and the narcissist.

In session, Ana could speak eloquently about how Moses mistreated her, even how he showed textbook signs of abuse: demanding to know where she was when they were apart; accusing her of infidelity; becoming so enraged and bereft that Ana felt compelled to apologize and soothe him, as though she were the one who had acted inappropriately. But at other times she lost this perspective. She felt she really *had* done something wrong and needed to earn back the affection of this man she'd only known for a few weeks, this man who could alternately be so doting and so cruel.

"You think you're the bad one because you've always thought that," I said while she was in one of these stormy, desperate states. "His abuse works because he's speaking to something that was planted in you a long time ago: the belief that you're rotten at the core."

"You can't prove that I'm *not* any more than I can prove that I *am*," she said.

"Who needs proof? Proof is overrated. I've known you a lot longer than Moses and I don't go out of my way to make you feel like shit. So, it can't just be you. It can't be a universal effect you have on people you're close to. Some of it must be coming from him."

When she ended things with Moses, Ana said she'd never broken up with someone before and that it was a strange, uncomfortable feeling. I mentioned Anders and she looked at me with a puzzled expression.

"Did I tell you that I broke up with him? I don't remember it that way. He'd iced me out so completely by that point. It was like I was tied to a dead body and I just cut the rope. What else was there to do? . . . He had already left me."

This turned out to be reflective of Ana's memory of all her romantic relationships, and of many close friendships as well. Even when she had been the one to end things—or when she took some action, like sleeping with someone else, that forced an ending—Ana never felt that she had been the one to leave. The other person was always the abandoner, which either left her inconsolable and empty, or justified some impulse such as jumping into another relationship or moving to a new place without leaving a forwarding address. Consciously inhabiting the role of the leaver for the first time with Moses presented the double-edged sword that comes with integrating a split, with moving from the infantile position where everyone is either all good or all bad to the place where people are a mix of both. On one hand it was empowering, marking a unique point in Ana's relational history in which she felt she had made a choice rooted in what she wanted and what she felt she deserved—a choice, no less, that favored solitude over being with someone, if that someone behaved like Moses had. On the other hand, the choice created the terrible sense of guilt that comes with a person recognizing that she is and has been responsible for her behavior, and has probably hurt other people. Ana had always felt helpless, ineffectual, and unloved—but now she was beginning to realize that perhaps others had, at times, felt abandoned by her.

Moses sent Ana a long text after the breakup, accusing her of seducing him. Now that they were finished, he said, he could see that this was actually the result he wanted: to be rid of her. Was *this* the difference between the borderline and the narcissist? Moses could only see himself as the one who leaves; Ana, until this moment, had seen herself only as the one who was left.

A month went by before Ana returned to the apps and matched with a man named Michael. They met, talked for three hours about Marx and Foucault, got drunk, and had sex. They began to see each other all the time. I wasn't sure what to make of this new person—Ana didn't talk about him the way she talked about past boyfriends. Their relationship was moving at a familiarly breakneck pace, punctuated by anecdotes of drunken chaos, and Ana recognized extreme thoughts ("I'm going to marry him someday," "I should never speak to him again") that caused her to worry that she was reenacting old scripts with a new scene partner. But I'd never before heard Ana use words like "thoughtful" and "patient" to describe a man she'd dated, past or present.

One night, about six weeks into their relationship, Ana told me Michael had seemed distracted during sex and had been unable to orgasm. She said this had never happened to her before and that she took it personally.

"I kept asking him, 'What's wrong, what happened?' And he kept saying, 'Nothing, nothing,' and I felt like he was lying to me. I said, 'Does this happen to you a lot? Do you not find me attractive? Are you gay?' And he said, 'No, no, no,' and he apologized, and said even though he didn't finish he had really enjoyed it. And I was feeling . . . I don't know how I was feeling. I said, 'Oh, you *like* this? Do you still like it if I do *this*?' And I kind of shoved him, and then I pinched him on the arm, and he laughed and said, 'No, not really,' and we were both kind of laughing and wrestling a bit and I kept saying, 'How about now? How about now?' And there was a knife on the coffee table from when we'd made food and I picked it up and held it to his throat and said, 'How about now?'"

She paused and looked at me. "I can tell by your face that you don't approve," she said.

I thought about this for a long time, to the point that Ana grew restless. "Do *you* approve?" I asked.

She smiled a toothy, nervous smile. "Of course I do. What a therapist thing to ask. I wouldn't have done it if I didn't approve."

I nodded slightly but otherwise said nothing.

"I didn't hurt him," she said. "I had no intention of hurting him. It was a joke."

"Oh," I said. "It was funny?"

Ana opened her mouth to speak but all that came out was a gasping sob, which surprised us both. "Of course not," she said after a moment. "I felt scared. Michael was so *understanding*, he said it was okay. But it wasn't okay. We kept wrestling and fighting and then had sex again. I felt like I was the only one in control but also completely *out* of control, like I was falling through a void. I think I wanted you to judge me today. I feel like I need judgment."

"How can I judge something I don't yet understand?"

"Yes, that's the thing. I say Michael is understanding but actually he doesn't understand. He didn't say, 'Hey, why are you doing this?' He didn't want to talk about it. He just said, 'It's okay.'"

"You kept pushing, looking for the boundary, and he kept yielding, and things deteriorated, until you both arrived at a scary place."

"I don't want to be this way. Do I have to stop seeing him?"

"A relationship has two people," I said. "You and Michael, you and me, you and Moses . . . anyone you've been involved with in the past. Even if it feels like you're the only one in control, you're not. You and I are used to discussing a question like, 'What does it mean that you're someone who would hold a knife to another person's throat?' Maybe we should also ask, 'What does it mean that Michael is someone who would have a knife held to his throat and not ask you to stop?'"

Ana arrived late to our next session. She said she'd had a good conversation with Michael, though I picked up a defensive tone from the start. At points she seemed to be trying to make me believe that she was seeing things in a balanced, distinctly non-borderline way. "I care a lot about him and would be very sad if we stopped seeing each other, but I wouldn't be devastated," she said in a clear voice. Then later she became fidgety and said she wanted to change the subject for fear that discussing her relationship with Michael with me would make her hate him.

On my commute home that evening I thought about this new relationship of Ana's. Part of me felt neutral about Michael, the same way I felt about every character a patient brings in when discussing the drama of her life. He was unreal to me, a facet of Ana's psychology that I was helping her make sense of on her own terms. I did not and would never know Michael; my contact was with Ana's internalization of him.

Beneath this lay a paternal feeling of which I was well aware: I wanted Ana to be with someone who I deemed, by some criteria, good enough. On this register I had positive feelings toward Michael. He seemed different from other men Ana had dated. Troubled, overly passive, yes, but not unkind. Of course, he didn't understand Ana yet (did I?), but he seemed like someone who could, someone who might genuinely want to understand her.

When I got home, Dawn asked me how my day was and I said, "Fine," in a way that implied I would be giving no elaboration. I felt miserly about the details of my day. It was in this moment that I discovered another feeling about Michael, one lying beneath my analytic neutrality and paternal concern. It was a feeling I can only describe as jealousy.

Ana's past boyfriends had been varying degrees of awful; I'd felt indignation toward them but also knew they would not dethrone me as the primary relationship in Ana's life. As my practice had expanded and, along with it, my experience of treating BPD, I had found that BPD patients would give me power and, if I rejected it outright, they would just find someone else to take it. I therefore had to handle this power differently than the others to whom they'd bestowed it in the past. But part of that difference had to be a willingness, at some point, to give the power back.

I didn't want to rule over Ana any longer. She was ready to grow beyond that state of dependence. Our relationship could survive a transition to something less hierarchical. I had to let these changes happen.

At our next session, Ana again arrived late.

"I don't know how to find my own thoughts lately," she began.

"How do you mean? Whose are you finding?"

"Well, when I'm here, I feel immediately closed off to you, and it's like Michael's inside my head. I keep wondering if you're trying to turn me against him, convince me to break up with him. So my thoughts are like Michael defending himself to you, even if you aren't saying anything."

"It's hard to think freely because if, say, a doubt about the relationship with Michael popped into your head, that feels like something you have to hide from me."

"I feel like I'm caught between the two of you and I'm getting smaller and smaller. I told Michael what you said about the other night, how neither of us put up a boundary and things deteriorated. And he said, 'Deteriorated? That's what people say when they're talking about Palestine or something.' I got so defensive, as though he were trying to convince me to leave *you*. I went on a whole rant about how important you are to me—I think I even said that dismissing something you said was the same as attacking me directly."

"It's a triangle," I said. I felt a palpable sense of relief—Ana was as ready to hear what I had to say as I was to tell her. "It's the shape of jealousy. It means there's always a third person who's not in the room, and the two people who *are* in the room can look out at the third instead of looking at each other. When you're here, you're mad at me and protective of Michael. When you're with Michael, it's inverted. So you're feeling all these mixed feelings, but never in the same place at the same time, where you'd have to reconcile them."

"I bring you in to speak for me a lot. 'Dr. Kriss said . . .' or 'Dr. Kriss wouldn't agree . . .' I say what's on my mind without admitting it's mine, and sometimes I actually forget whether or not it is mine. And then Michael gets defensive and the next thing I know we're having a debate about you, who's not there and who he's never met, instead of talking about us."

Over the coming weeks Ana expressed variations on the theme of fearing that she was losing herself within the relationship with Michael. Sometimes she was angry with me, or him, or herself; often she appeared dissociated and dulled. Then, suddenly, she would show up one day lucid and bright, often after spending a night by herself. "I know I need more alone time," she would say, though days in which she actually carved out such time came few and far between.

Ana started sending me emails with subject lines like, "Why am I rancid?"

Since I have a more accurate and historical recollection of abandonment and abuse, there's a sense of familiarity which is terrifying in a new way. I used to feel like this all the time but would tell myself it was the first time, or the worst it had ever been. Now I see how much of a pattern it all is and how deep it goes. I'm not just afraid of being abandoned by a person but by myself, I'm scared I won't just lose a relationship but my mind. I feel like we've worked so hard but during times like this, I remember the "old me" is still here.

Around this time Ana recounted a dream: "I'm on the beach surrounded by puppies and my father is with me. He instructs me to take the puppies one by one into the water and drown them, and I do it." She paused, moving her gaze from the floor to me. "Did you know this would happen? Is this progress? Now I can see my whole horrible history laid out behind me, how my father controlled me, turned me against my own nature, primed me to be controlled by future men. So, what? Can I never have a functional relationship?

What is the point of our therapy, beyond helping me see I am broken beyond repair?"

Ana and I understood that these questions were, at least to some degree, hyperbolic. She had derived tangible benefits from our therapy; on a day-to-day basis Ana felt little doubt that she was better off now than she'd been two years prior. Ana also appreciated, when in a less distressed state of mind, that her frustration came from a part of her that assumed a romantic relationship had to be the defining feature of her life, even as she was spending time—more than ever before—entertaining the thought that this might not be the case. She still toyed with the idea of returning to school, though she admitted that the tumult of her relationship with Michael—and Moses before him, and Anders before him—kept distracting her from taking steps toward doing so.

And yet. Why *were* we still doing this? Because it helped Ana? Because she kept showing up to my office? How would we know when to stop?

I couldn't say what the point of therapy was for Ana because I wasn't Ana. This frustrated her, but it also frightened me. I had to trust that she would figure things out for herself, and not in the paternalistic sense of, "I know the right answer but it will build character to find it on your own." This was less certain, more free. I didn't know if seeing Michael was a good idea, or what Ana should do with her life. I believed in the work we were doing. As for where it would lead . . . wasn't that what people called faith?

"You're here on time," I said as Ana sat down. We were nearing the end of our second year.

"I am," she said. "I know I've been late a lot recently."

"True," I said.

"It's almost unbelievable, when I think about it. I used to wish I could never leave here. Do you remember when I asked if I could sleep under the couch?"

"Now it's as if you're trying to limit our time together."

"I've been very angry and very confused. I cry a lot. I try to keep more things to myself. It's hard, between you and Michael, to do that." She smiled and I had no idea what it meant. "Have you ever seen *The Thing*? Michael and I watched it last night."

"I have. It's actually one of my favorite films."

"Really? I loved it. I think it's one of my favorites now, too."

We sat in silence for a while and I started thinking about *The Thing*. An alien organism infiltrates a research station in Antarctica, preying on the twelve men working there. When it devours its victims it also produces perfect copies of them, and consequently, it becomes impossible to know who is a person and who is a thing. No one is even sure if they are themselves a copy or not. In perhaps the most famous scene, Kurt Russell's character, R. J. MacReady, is trying to determine who is still human by dipping a searing hot wire into a sample of each person's blood: if the wire fizzles, it indicates the blood of a human. Everyone is in a big room together, some tied up, all eyeing one another with paranoia and fear. First, MacReady tests the blood of a man called Windows. Windows leans forward, sweat dripping down his brow, petrified until the moment the wire fizzles, and then he's flooded with relief. Then MacReady says to the room, "Now I'll show you what I already know," and tests his own blood without batting an eye.

That's when you realize that MacReady is the only one in the movie who truly believes that he's a human being. Everyone else hopes that they are, but they aren't sure. They don't trust their thoughts or memories—not completely, not enough that they aren't open to the possibility that when the wire hits the blood, it will reveal they're something else. That's why MacReady is the hero: it's so rare to know who you are.

"You know, you've never asked me," Ana said, stirring me from my reverie.

"Never asked you what?"

"Why I didn't kill myself."

She glanced out the window, perhaps recalling the day she'd threatened to jump out of it. "I know I used to talk about it a lot. I thought about it even more. More than I ever told you, especially this past year. You must have known on some level. But you never asked why I didn't do it."

Sometimes I would daydream about receiving a call that Ana was in the hospital. I wondered what it would be like to visit her in that kind of place, the locked psych ward. So, she was right—on some level I had known.

"I guess I assumed you had your reasons," I said.

She laughed, and in that laughter started to cry. "I knew you would say something like that," she said.

Sometimes I run into my psychologist neighbor around town. She's friendly and we continue to have little to say to each other. I don't feel angry when I see her—now, I feel something more like pity. Because when I see her, or anyone else who rolls their eyes at the borderline, who disparages it as difficult or crazy, who wants, for the sake of managing their own anxiety, to believe that there is nothing we can learn from it, I think of what Ana said next.

"I was a mystery to myself. I can't explain how terrifying that feels. I wanted to die, at so many different times for so many different reasons . . . but I felt that I should know who I was before deciding to act. If I knew myself and still wanted to die, then I would know that I had tried. That it was a choice. But I felt I owed it to myself to wait."

DIFFUSION

1973–2011

A s the *DSM-III* was being prepared in 1970s America, the view of psychological life was hazy, like looking into a mirror coated in dust. Mainstream psychoanalysis had become rigid, dogmatic, and authoritarian; it was hard to see anyone clearly. The factions forming across psychoanalysis, psychiatry, and psychology did not try to learn from the past or from each other; instead, they began to carve out proprietary domains, often defined in terms of their opposition to other factions. When it came to borderline individuals, the result of this balkanization was a splintering of knowledge about their experience and history that made understanding harder, not easier, and did little to discourage unhelpful treatments—in some cases, it allowed strange new ways of abusing borderline patients to flourish.

After the *DSM-III*'s publication in 1980, the dirty mirror was not so much cleaned as shattered, broken into different shards. Each represented an attempt to grapple with the borderline from a different school of thought; each ran in untouching parallel to the others.

One shard concerned the case of Shirley Mason, born in 1923 in Minnesota. The details of her early life have been much debated, and there are few definitive facts: we know that she was raised by strict Protestant parents; that her mother, described by a neighbor as "witch-like," may or may not have been diagnosed with schizophrenia.[1] We know that Mason, beginning in adolescence, suffered from episodes of intense emotional overwhelm and dissociation. As a young adult she traveled listlessly around the Midwest, seeking treatment at the University of Nebraska's medical center in her twenties. There she met Dr. Cornelia Burwell Wilbur, one of the few women in the center's psychiatry department. In 1949, Wilbur and Mason met again in New York—the former had moved there to begin analytic training and the latter to attend graduate school at Columbia University—and they commenced a course of psychoanalysis.

Before long, Wilbur made what she believed was a startling discovery: Mason's slight, unassuming frame appeared to contain not one but many personalities. According to Wilbur, Mason would slip in and out of different "selves" at different times, shifts often catalyzed by stressful events. Each personality possessed its own name, disposition, and interests, and held limited knowledge of the other personalities or of Mason as a whole.

For decades, academic journals rebuffed as absurd and unscientific Wilbur's attempts to publish on her claims of discovering sixteen distinct personalities living inside of Mason.[2] Wilbur therefore decided to approach a journalist, Florence Schreiber, to write up the case as a book for general audiences. Mason was renamed "Sybil," which also served as the title of the book, published in 1973. In 1976 a TV movie adaptation followed, starring Sally Field. These works brought Wilbur's term, multiple personality disorder (MPD), not only into the public consciousness but the professional one. A concept that had barely existed before 1973 exploded in prevalence over the ensuing decade.[3] MPD was included in the *DSM-III*, four years before any paper by Wilbur on the subject was accepted for publication by a peer-reviewed scientific journal.[4]

Two questions come to mind. First: How was it possible that a twentieth-century doctor saw Shirley Mason's condition and thought that she was looking at something new? As depicted in Schreiber's book, Mason's rapid mood swings, episodes of dissociation, and chronic difficulties maintaining jobs and relationships read like a case study you might find in the work of Otto Kernberg, Sándor Ferenczi, Sigmund Freud, or even Thomas Sydenham. Why didn't Wilbur believe any of this history was relevant to explaining Mason's experience? There has been much speculation about Wilbur's motives over the years. Some have cast her as an eclectic genius; others point to pressures she must have felt to succeed as a woman in a male-dominated field, still others to more crass ambitions for fame and fortune.

Ultimately these factors served as the match to underlying kindling. Wilbur had been trained in the milieu of midcentury American psychiatry, which held no space for the borderline between neurosis and psychosis—"never the twain shall meet," as Robert Knight wrote of the mainstream psychoanalytic attitude around the time Wilbur was training as an analyst. She concocted a new explanation to an old problem because she had little exposure to the knowledge that might have illuminated a common thread going back thousands of years. Perhaps this led Wilbur to overemphasize a salacious symptom rather than seeing it as part of a bigger picture—perhaps, as her sharpest critics suggest, she actively created for Mason the narrative of multiple selves as a way to make sense of something neither she nor Mason understood.

The second and more important question: How did Wilbur manage to permanently etch a diagnosis into psychiatry's bible? That she diagnosed Mason with multiple personalities is only of significance to the history of BPD or anything else because of how far that diagnosis spread. It began with *Sybil*: written in oily prose by Schreiber, the book sold millions of copies, and Sally Field won an Emmy for her portrayal of Mason. But, as ever, this was no coincidence. *Sybil* inflamed public imagination because it emerged at just the right time, in a kind of theoretical vortex.

American psychoanalysis was quickly falling out of fashion, and once *Sybil* had made Wilbur something of a celebrity, the story of the long-standing rejection of her work by her colleagues sounded to the general public like the old guard trying to censor a modern voice. Modern, especially, in terms of how the book and film depicted psychotherapy sessions in which Wilbur connected Mason's multiple personalities to her supposed traumatic childhood. Public interest in early trauma was unprecedently high in the mid-1970s, thanks in large part to the attention drawn to it by the women's liberation movement—an evolution from the previous decade's countercultural-ism, which had been broadly infused with anti-psychiatry sentiments and now regarded ego psychology as patriarchal and sexist.

Perhaps above all, Wilbur's diagnostic label became famous just as psychiatry's dependence on diagnostic labels reached its height. The *DSM-III*, which was being prepared amid the *Sybil* craze, cate-gorized illness by symptoms rather than underlying causes or theo-ries—and in the wake of a best-selling book and popular movie, the symptoms of MPD started popping up everywhere. Patients began reporting experiences of having multiple selves in alarming numbers; if psychiatry hadn't made room for these patients in its diagnostic bible, it would have had to cede authority over them.

MPD persists as a diagnosis today, renamed dissociative identity disorder (DID) in 1994 with the publication of the *DSM-IV*, but otherwise largely unchanged from its 1980 origins as a systemati-zation of Schreiber's famous book about Mason.[5] David Spiegel, an American psychiatrist who led the renaming committee, explained the rationale once in an interview: "'Multiple personality' carries with it the implication that they really have more than one person-ality. . . . Dissociative identity disorder implies that the problem is fragmentation of identity, not that you really are twelve people. That you have, not more than one, but less than one personality."[6] The extent to which one finds this reasoning compelling may come down to a matter of taste—justifying a name is not the same thing as demonstrating its value.

DID remains a controversial diagnosis: it has been sensational-ized in countless more films and television shows, and placed at the center of class-action lawsuits against therapists by former patients alleging that they were coerced into believing that they had this disorder while in a state of vulnerability. Debate often revolves around the question of whether DID or multiple personalities are "real"—a question that is, I think, long since irrelevant. Can we ever say that the naming of things, whether through diagnosis or some other form of labeling, is real? The relevant point is that Wilbur, and then others following her ideas from greater positions of power, made a categorical error. Rather than viewing multiple personalities as a metaphor for what it feels like to live on the borderline, they took it literally—and in so doing declared it to be its own thing. It's unclear if we can ever fully return from such a rigid and highly publicized delineation. Whether Wilbur induced Mason's perception of multiple selves or not, she gave it the stamp of authority.

Diagnosis is not passive: it changes how we think of someone and, crucially, how we treat them. In Mason's case, Wilbur gave her a label that suggested a new condition, a strange and groundbreaking enigma that only Wilbur could decipher. It bound doctor and patient to each other for the rest of their lives. After their formal analysis ended, the two remained in constant contact: Mason relocated to Kentucky when Wilbur took up an academic position there; Wilbur loaned Mason the money to put a down payment on a house. When Wilbur was diagnosed with Parkinson's disease in 1991, Mason moved into her former doctor's home to care for her until her death the following year. Mason died six years later of breast cancer, which, after learning of the diagnosis, she opted not to treat.

Haku was first referred to my practice by a psychologist, Sarah, who worked at the counseling center of the college Haku attended. When we spoke on the phone, Sarah described Haku as a cisgender Japanese American man who had withdrawn completely from social life. He had stopped going to class and his roommates reported that Haku spent all waking and sleeping hours squeezed underneath his bed with less than two feet of headroom, accompanied by a blanket, a stuffed panda, and his laptop. Sarah said that, based on her limited assessment, Haku was either severely depressed or experiencing some kind of psychotic break, or perhaps both. The school wanted him to take a medical leave and go home to his parents. This would leave open the possibility of him returning to school in the future—otherwise he was likely to flunk out and would be forcibly removed from campus. Sarah asked if I would be open to a consultation with Haku.

"He won't get into any details with me about what's going on and keeps saying he needs someone who specializes in 'dissociation,'" she said. "He definitely needs to be in treatment, plus the school would need documentation from a psychologist clearing Haku to come back next semester."

I said I would be happy to meet with Haku if he wanted to meet with me, but could make no promises about where treatment would lead or, if he left school now, whether he would be ready to return a few months later.

"That's fine, that's fine," Sarah said, not attempting to hide her relief. "We just don't know what else to do for him. Also, his parents will want to talk to you. He refused to give me permission to speak to them, but said he would for someone who knows about dissociation. I'll be honest, I'm so confused by this case."

After receiving written consent from Haku, mediated through Sarah, I arranged to speak to his mother. It was unusual for me to do this before meeting with an adult patient, though I understood that Haku's parents—who would be paying for his treatment—were likely not used to thinking of their son as an adult, as he had only recently turned eighteen.

His mother presented a new picture: Haku was a white transgender man with a long history of extreme and impulsive behavior beginning around age twelve. Haku had recently, on his eighteenth birthday, legally changed his name to that of a character from the

Hayao Miyazaki film *Spirited Away*. His mother said Haku had a history of suicide attempts, destruction of property, and running away from home, sometimes disappearing for weeks at a time without contact. The family had tried various forms of treatment over the past six years, from individual and family psychotherapies to inpatient hospitalizations, from monthslong therapeutic wilderness schools to medication. Haku had been diagnosed at various points with attention-deficit/hyperactivity disorder, bipolar disorder, and autism.

"Do you want me to *really* get into it?" she asked, referring to her son's history, after we had been speaking for about half an hour.

"I think I should speak to Haku first," I said.

We met via video conference, me in my office and Haku wedged tightly under his dorm room bed. On my screen, somewhat grainy from low light, I saw a round, pale face with small, deep-set eyes and a dense frizz of dark brown hair. I was immediately struck by how plausible it was for this person to be either of the versions with which I'd been presented so far: he could be trans or cis, white or Japanese. Framed by LED lights strung around his cramped living space, I saw in Haku's face sadness, fear, and a vague sense of menace.

"Hi," he said in a high-pitched voice that did not seem entirely natural.

"Hi," I said. "Haku?"

He furrowed his brow and stared at me through the screen for several seconds.

"We don't know what this is," he finally said. "We saw it in the calendar, so we clicked the link."

A third picture emerged in bits and pieces. Haku was neither cis nor trans, but nonbinary. He was neither Japanese nor white, but nonracial. He was not even Haku—he said that he had heard the name before but did not identify with it. Presently, he said, he did not know his name. He referred to his parents as "the parents" and also said that they were not really his parents, because they had not created him.

"I know they birthed the host body, we understand biology," he said. "But each of us came from different places. I was born in a forest of light and my mother is a stone castle."

"I see," I said, though of course I didn't see. "Does this have anything to do with dissociation? I was told you wanted to talk to someone who knew about dissociation."

"*I* don't know about that," he said. "That must have been one of the others. But yes, we hear talk of that word. One of the others has said that we have dissociative identity disorder. Am I saying that right? Things have become much easier since we learned that we are not a person."

"What are you, then?"

"We are a system."

Over the coming weeks, I learned more about this system, though it was complicated and contradictory. Haku told me that he was filled with many selves, not all of which were human or could speak. (I have elected to use masculine pronouns to refer to Haku, as he most often identified as a man in our sessions.) This could come across as floridly psychotic, yet there was a coherence to his descriptions that felt different from patients I'd worked with who were in the grips of psychosis. A lot of the imagery he used was drawn from Japanese anime and video games with which I happened to be familiar, and the stories he told of his different selves sometimes followed their plots beat for beat. Most of the time, Haku spoke using the eerie first-person plural, though at times he would slip into the singular—on more than one occasion I watched him catch himself and self-consciously snap back into the former mode. It's not that I thought he was faking it, not any more than I think Shirley Mason was. It seemed more that Haku *wanted* to have multiple personalities, even if that meant he had to force himself and others to believe in it.

But why? Most obviously, it was because the act of dividing himself meant that no single piece held the memory of the whole. As with any split—in this case, the supposed splitting of Haku's personality—the good was separated, and thus protected, from the bad. Specifically, Haku said the system spared him from facing "the trauma," an unspecified event from the past that no part of him was interested in discussing.

"We've read that the goal of treating DID is integration, but we don't want to integrate."

"What *do* you want?" I asked.

He considered this. "To be left alone."

I felt this to be the most unambiguously genuine thing that I'd heard Haku say.

"Do you want to go back to school?" I asked, which had nominally been the point of us meeting in the first place—to establish a relationship so that, in a few months' time, I might verify his mental fitness to resume academic life.

"No," he said. "The parents want us to go to school, and we need them for financial support. If I could find a job, I would drop out of school for good. . . . *We* would save up enough money to buy a shitty car and drive out to California."

"Oh? What's in California?"

A sudden guardedness descended. "A friend," he said.

More weeks and more sessions passed. It became clear that, beginning several months ago, not long after starting school, Haku had begun a relationship of some sort with a person he'd met online. This person shared many of Haku's common interests, including gaming and anime, and also disclosed a history of similar behavioral issues. One day, the friend asked Haku if he had ever considered that he had DID. Haku said he knew nothing about it, beyond vague references in popular culture. From there, a process that I can only describe as indoctrination commenced, as Haku's friend introduced to him the concept of a "system," detailed how a system worked, and suggested that each of Haku's emotional states represented a different self. The friend also introduced the idea of "the trauma" as some singular moment in Haku's life that had broken him into a million pieces. At one point, Haku shared text messages with me in which the friend explicitly instructed him on how to deceive his parents and therapists so that they wouldn't try to "reintegrate" him.

"Do you think your friend has your best interests in mind?" I asked at one point.

"Yes," Haku said.

"I'm not so sure. They have a story about who you are that doesn't make a lot of sense to me. Most people who have had a lot of problems throughout their lives can't source them back to one big event. It's usually a combination of things that builds up gradually. It's the gradual buildup that can make it hard to keep track of why things are the way they are—it can also make simple narratives like 'the trauma' appealing. But that doesn't make it real."

"Are you saying my system isn't real?"

I took a moment to consider this question. "Honestly, who am I to say? It's not an *objective* system. You don't literally have people and creatures inside of you, or lots of little brains inside your skull. It's a mental system, an emotional system, and no one has access to that but you."

"Okay," he said.

"I'm not trying to convince you of anything. But I do find myself wondering why you wanted to see me in the first place. Why did you request to see an expert on dissociation? You say you don't want to go back to school, you say you don't want to change. Why bring me into your life at all?"

For several moments Haku wore a strange, forced smile on his face. Then he let it drop and seemed, perhaps for the first time since we'd met, relaxed.

"It's very hard for me to trust people. I don't trust the parents. I don't trust the school. I trust my friend. But . . ."

"You wondered if someone like me might see things differently. That maybe if you found a therapist you trusted, they could help you."

"We've had a lot of therapists. Some were nice, others not so much. I don't know."

"Maybe it feels like you have to choose. You want your friend's love, but you know on some level they don't understand. You want me to understand, but you know on some level . . ."

I didn't quite know where I was going with this. The fake smile returned to Haku's face.

Within the next few weeks our treatment ended. His mother said she couldn't afford to have Haku keep seeing me if we weren't headed toward him returning to school.

"He needs to see someone," I said to her on the phone. "He's very confused right now. He's stuck on a particular idea about who he is. If he doesn't have anyone to help him question it, things could get a lot worse."

"I understand," she said. She sounded tired. "Probably things will get worse. That's been the story. I'd say I want him to reach the point where we could hospitalize him, but that's never helped, either."

She ended the call. I emailed Haku to say that, while I understood he couldn't afford to work with me anymore, as a legal adult he was free to look for treatment elsewhere. I included information for some low-fee clinics in the area.

"No need," he replied later the same day. "We'll be in California soon. Thanks for listening."

The next mirror shard came from psychiatry. The field's emphasis on medication, beginning in the 1980s, placed BPD outside its purview—the condition had never, under any of its names, responded well to biological intervention. This did not mean that, post-*DSM-III*, psychiatrists began to accurately diagnose and refer out borderline patients as they passed through their offices. More likely, psychiatrists would misdiagnose these patients and then regard them as difficult. At least as far back as the nineteenth century, we have records of doctors like W. Tyler Smith expressing frustration at patients whose illness did not conform to treatment. Psychiatrists of the 1980s, severed from the lessons of psychoanalysis on why history repeats itself, began to repeat Smith's errors and frustrations. As psychiatric training focused more on disorders it could effectively treat, psychiatrists developed an implicit bias toward diagnosing patients with those disorders.[7] When patients didn't respond to treatment, they were marked as having an "atypical" or "treatment-resistant" case.

In at least one instance, the *DSM-III* committee created a diagnosis from whole cloth in its effort to make sense of epidemiological data severed from theory and history. We find in that text, and all subsequent editions of the *DSM*, a curious condition known as cyclothymic disorder (CD).[8] It was formalized to acknowledge the large number of patients who seemed to show features of bipolar disorder—episodic peaks of mania and nadirs of depression—yet whose peaks never qualified as fully manic, nor the nadirs as fully depressive, with episodes that were often faster and blurrier than expected. CD seemed to defy what bipolarity was supposed to be, yet the psychiatric establishment seemed unable to consider that the bipolar framework might not apply here. No matter that CD patients often did not respond to the same treatments that tended to help other bipolar cases, namely mood-stabilizing drugs like lithium; or that while bipolar disorder had been found consistently in the population for as long as data had been collected, CD had mysteriously leapt from rare to very common in the late 1970s; or that while bipolar disorder seemed to be evenly distributed across men and women, CD was mostly diagnosed in women. It was and is a further diffusion of the borderline, which can be found spread indiscriminately throughout the *DSM*, from CD in the category of mood disorders, to DID in dissociative disorders, to BPD, HPD, and NPD in personality disorders.

Terms like "atypical" and "treatment-resistant" are still bandied about in psychiatric circles today with a casual cruelty. The assumption is that the diagnosis, and by extension the doctor who bestows it, is inviolate: "treatment-resistant depression" suggests that the patient must be depressed but for some reason is being stubborn about getting better. But what if she is something else, or something more? Then it would be the diagnosis that is wrong, as well as the corresponding treatment—perhaps even the doctor. This is a tough reality to consider if you are working in a discipline bound to a text like the *DSM* and interventions like pills.* Once a patient doesn't fit into the model, there is nowhere left to go.

The last quarter of the twentieth century saw a growing number of non-MD professionals working in mental health—clinical psychologists and, by the turn of the twenty-first century, legions of master's-level social workers and counselors. Many of these professionals followed psychiatrists in adopting the *DSM-III* as a guide to conceptualizing and diagnosing illness. But they were in need of their own approach to treatment, a psychological intervention to rival the biological. What would fill the void left by the categorical rejection of psychoanalysis? Which piece of the broken mirror would these new authorities inhabit?

American psychologist Albert Ellis had been working since the 1950s on a so-called rational therapy that sought, in the vein of the ur-therapist Galen of Pergamon, to teach patients how to identify and logically challenge irrational feelings and beliefs.[9] Meanwhile, in the early 1960s, psychiatrist Aaron Beck began earnestly developing his "cognitive therapy" as a way to treat depression, specifically by helping patients to reframe negative thoughts about the self, the world, and the future.[10] Beck, who was analytically trained, had been excommunicated from his professional community for this

---

*It is worth noting that several of my patients diagnosed with BPD have taken psychiatric medication to good effect. I encourage patients who are interested in medication to explore the option—specifically, as a supplement to psychotherapy that works best when prescribed by a psychiatrist whom they find thoughtful and trustworthy.

work, especially because of his interest in briefer treatments than the yearslong analyses typical of mid-twentieth-century America, as well as his interest in conducting research on the effectiveness of psychotherapy in general. Beck and Ellis, working independently in the shadow of mainstream psychiatry, would in the 1980s serve as driving forces behind the rise of cognitive-behavioral therapy (CBT)—the successor to psychoanalysis's vacant throne.

The imperial conquest of CBT would eventually be so complete, not just in the United States but across the world, that in the twenty-first century many psychologists, social workers, counselors, and members of the general public would regard it as synonymous with the word "psychotherapy," just as psychoanalysis had been for much of the century prior. This ascent occurred not only in the tumult of post-*DSM-III* psychiatry but amid a broader cognitive revolution in the field of academic psychology. The Freudian metaphor of archaeology as model for the human condition was systematically replaced by a more contemporary one: the computer. The mind was no longer dense strata, with some layers accessible near the surface and others buried far beneath. Understanding the mind, in turn, was no longer a matter of plumbing the depths to unearth that which had been lost to consciousness. Instead, the mind was now seen as a machine, sophisticated but nevertheless operating according to the basic algorithm of computational science: input, processing, and output.

Just as we often evoke psychoanalytic language without realizing it ("Don't be so defensive!"), so too has the mind-as-machine concept entered daily speech in an insidious way. "I need to process this," we say, though for the late twentieth-century cognitive-behaviorist, "processing" carried a very specific meaning. The idea was that people, like a computer, think and act according to rules and logic; that we are fundamentally rational beings. Emotional difficulties were therefore the result of faulty thinking that must be corrected, or conditioned behaviors that must be reconditioned. From this vantage there was little room for the psychotic core, for contradiction or ambivalence: the new metaphor conferred an implicit assumption that, as with machines, a healthy human is an optimized human. We should want to be well, to be productive, to be happy. So it is little wonder that as countless therapists learned to deliver these new treatments to patients—now usually called "clients" within the CBT framework, which, depending on one's point of view, could be seen as an attempt to make mental health services either more egalitarian or more businesslike—and as researchers produced a vast literature of empirical studies to validate CBT's efficacy, therapist and researcher alike kept running into the problem of the borderline.

Beck had been highly critical of the notion of personality disorders: he felt they were too nebulous to define—and to therefore treat or research—and objected to their inclusion in the *DSM-III*.[11] Ellis, meanwhile, was disinterested in the very notion of the self: he saw the word "personality" as an embodiment of the rigid self-narratives that his therapeutic approach tried to help people overcome.

CBT should be understood in this paradoxical context—that is, of stemming from founders who, through the metaphor of machines, were trying to create something more humane than what American ego psychology had become. A computer does not need to be programmed with a sense of what its function is: a piece of chess software isn't trying to win, it's just following rules to a logical outcome. So, too, does CBT presume people to be naturally self-driven and self-correcting, whether or not we speak of some underlying sense of purpose, personality, or self. Trying to understand how a person came to be the way they are, from this point of view, is as unnecessary as trying to find the specific software engineer who programmed your buggy computer. What matters is assessing the current, manifest problem and treating it directly.

All this rests on a crucial assumption: that the removal of a symptom, like fixing a software bug, will restore the individual to a previously healthy state. A person is well, then becomes afflicted with depression, then his depression is removed, then he is well again. As a reaction to American ego psychology—which found a way to treat anyone and everyone as ill—this approach released a breath of fresh air into the stale musk of the analyst's consulting room. But, like psychoanalysis, CBT could be drawn to its own dehumanizing extreme—an extreme that characterizes much of the conversation around psychological issues in the modern day.

For starters, what is a healthy state? What do we mean when we say we want to be happy, or live our "best" life? Are we supposed to be completely free of anything that might resemble a symptom as found in the exhaustive bullet list of the *DSM*, or perhaps free of anything at all that feels unpleasant—of anxiety, sadness, fear, or anger? Even less clear is how to consider someone who has never known this presumed original healthy state. Someone who has grown up around chaos and madness; someone who defies Beck and Ellis's contention that talking about "the self" is superfluous because everybody has one.

My view of the CBT establishment should not be construed as an indictment of all its practitioners. I have known many cognitive-behavioral therapists to be thoughtful and flexible, resisting the extreme and dogmatic aspects of the movement as the best psychoanalysts did and continue to do—and as do those working from any theoretical perspective. But the cognitive-behavior perspective has running through it an emphasis on order and category (inherited from the *DSM*) and on rational, logical processes (inherited from the cognitive revolution) that has rendered it unsuitable for BPD, or anyone lost in the diffusion of modern diagnoses. Just as the BPD diagnosis entered the new mainstream via the *DSM-III*, those who suffered from it were again set adrift—either mistreated or untreated by the new breed of medication-oriented psychiatrists on one side and CBT-trained psychotherapists on the other.

"At the start of every session he would ask me to rate my mood over the past week on a scale of one to ten," a patient of mine once described of her previous experience with CBT. "One day I said, 'Every number. I have been every number this week.' And that was true, but I also wanted him to acknowledge me in a specific way. I understand now that I wanted to break the structure of the session. I felt like he hated me and I thought that, if I could make him deviate from the formula, it would mean I'd done something special and won him over. He stared at me, holding his pen over his pad of paper, and he said, 'So, should we call that a five?' I didn't go back after that."

Among the scattered shards of multiple personalities, biological psychiatry, and the rise of cognitive-behaviorism, by the late 1980s conditions were ripe for the next great synthesizer. Someone who would pick up the torch once held by Galen, Freud, and most recently Kernberg; someone who would try to address the borderline problem while adhering to the professional and cultural strictures of the present day.

American psychologist Marsha Linehan would do all of this and more: she would draw from psychoanalysis, Christianity, and Buddhism while cleverly packaging these strands as compatible, even synonymous, with cognitive science. She would make BPD a household term and help shape our modern concept of mental health as something that can be taught through skills training and meditation apps. She would also be the first since Melanie Klein to draw on a specific source of knowledge and incorporate it into her view of borderline phenomena: the firsthand experience of being a patient.

In 1987, Linehan began publishing on a treatment that she'd developed, dialectical behavior therapy (DBT)—the first psychological treatment specifically created for people diagnosed with BPD. If one is not considering the history of its creator, defining DBT can be surprisingly difficult. It is marked by contradiction and paradox: a flexible theory executed through rigid technique; a structured approach marked by loose boundaries; a cognitive-behavioral therapy that rejects basic assumptions of CBT; a compassionate and effective treatment that has helped to drive stigma for the past thirty years. Nevertheless, I will try to define DBT as an abstraction before unpacking where it came from and where it has taken us.

At its core, DBT is rooted in Linehan's belief that people with BPD are suffering from a "dialectical failure"—that is, they cannot hold contradictory truths in mind at the same time.[12] This was, in some ways, using new language to describe the old concept of splitting. Linehan even used that word, noting that one of the major dialectics of life was appreciating that people have both positive and negative qualities, and that you cannot reduce things to all good or all bad without severely distorting your sense of reality. But she placed even greater value on a different dialectic, one that had roots in both psychoanalytic and existential sources: the tension between acceptance and change.

Linehan astutely pointed out that people with BPD often felt like they hated themselves, and in their hatred rendered personal change impossible. They were always trying to turn into someone else, to escape, and when their sudden and often extreme attempts at doing so—switching cities, jobs, friends, partners, adopting a new lifestyle or religion, giving up or taking up substances—inevitably receded and revealed that they were still themselves, they hated the new person they thought they had become. DBT addressed this phenomenon through a philosophy of "radical acceptance," in which the present had to be tolerated in order to allow the possibility of change in the future.[13] Therapists, too, were expected to model the paradoxical dialogue that their patients struggled with: to walk the line between enabling their patient's behavior (accepting the present without encouraging change) and judging it as unhealthy (encouraging change without accepting the present); to find a way to embrace patients as they were while simultaneously pushing them to be different—or, perhaps more accurately, pushing them to *behave* differently.

"I have never been interested in borderline personality disorder as a 'disorder' in itself," Linehan wrote in her 2020 memoir, *Building a Life Worth Living*. "I have never targeted that. I target suicidal behavior, out-of-control behavior. I don't think of myself as treating a disorder. I treat a set of behaviors that gets turned into a disorder by others."[14]

In many respects this was patently true, and we will see the origins and consequences of Linehan's behavioral focus in short order. It is also true that she largely adopted the nomenclature of BPD in order to appease the psychiatric and psychological authorities that demanded adherence to names that could be found in the *DSM-III*. But, from the start, DBT was *not* only interested in behavior. Linehan also placed emotion, particularly the struggle to *regulate* emotion, at the center of BPD. The overwhelming nature of feelings was to Linehan both a driving cause of the behavioral side of the disorder and the part of borderline experience that patients found most distressing.

Emotion was a curious focus for a researcher trained almost exclusively in cognitive-behaviorism. Beck had framed psychological suffering, especially depression, as a matter of thought distortion: first you think, "I'm worthless," and then, as a kind of by-product, you feel sad. As his and Ellis's ideas expanded to touch nearly every aspect of mental illness and health, the primacy of thought remained. But Linehan said the opposite. Though she took pains to distinguish herself from Kernberg's transference-based approach and the broader analytic tradition he represented, in this respect she had more in common with him than most of her CBT colleagues. Emotion—the overflowing, unbounded discharge of raw psychic energy—lay at the heart of borderline experience. In fact, cognition played a relatively small role for patients who so often moved from unbearable feeling to impulsive action, seeming to skip over thought entirely.

DBT in theory was flexible and pluralistic; in practice it was rigid, or at least was presented as such. Linehan outlined a specific protocol that demanded a substantial buy-in from doctors and patients alike: to receive DBT one had to enroll in a comprehensive regimen of individual therapy, group therapy, and intermittent coaching sessions by phone. DBT therapy groups followed a prescribed curriculum with accompanying homework assignments; various protocols, especially around assessing and reducing suicidal thoughts and behaviors, had to be carried out in a particular way and at particular times. This is why many professionals today advertise their services as "DBT-informed": there is debate over whether one can claim to practice DBT if they are not following Linehan's model to the letter.

Some of this rigidity came out of how DBT rose in prominence. As a young researcher, Linehan knew that her work—a novel treatment created by a woman and focused on a notoriously female disorder—would only have a chance at being taken seriously if her methods stood beyond reproach. During the 1980s and '90s, this meant constructing clinical trials modeled after pharmaceutical science, in which experimental and control groups were compared through statistical analysis.

The gold standard of this approach, known as the randomized controlled trial (RCT), was a far cry from the case studies of psychoanalysis, where the psychology of a single patient would be laid out as evidence for a given theory or treatment. The case study benefited from depth—it offered nuanced data about how a single person engaged in treatment and changed over time, potentially years—but suffered from poor controls: in any given case it was impossible to say whether the documented changes would have also occurred with a different therapist or kind of therapy, or if they would have happened spontaneously anyway, as there was no doppelgänger to whom the patient could be compared. RCTs took an inverse approach: patients would be randomly assigned to groups as a way of controlling for individual factors, so that differences between groups could be more confidently attributed to the experimental condition—such as receiving DBT versus some other treatment. What was lost was the depth and texture of the real world: in order to maintain laboratory-like conditions, RCTs usually required strict inclusion and exclusion criteria, forcing patients into firm categories and, therefore, favoring patients who conformed to those categories. These studies also, by design, put a hard ceiling on following up with patients, usually a year or less, limiting what could be inferred about the long-term effects of any treatment being evaluated.

Without a doubt, much of DBT's success—it is now the most prevalent treatment for BPD in the world, and by some metrics one of the most successfully evangelized psychotherapies of the modern era—can be attributed to how well Linehan played the game of research academia.[15] But even if we poke holes in her empirical studies—or in the very notion of RCTs as a useful way to measure things as complex as mental health and psychotherapy—it is hard to deny the value of certain DBT ideas once you've been exposed to them.

Beyond its core concept of radical acceptance, DBT's greatest innovation was the introduction of ancient concepts from Zen Buddhism into the psychotherapist's repertoire. Interest in meditation practices from East and South Asia had been growing in the United States as part of various countercultural movements beginning in the 1960s—the term "mindfulness" entered the Western lexicon by way of Vietnamese monk Thích Nhất Hạnh's best-selling 1975 book, *The Miracle of Mindfulness*.[16] But the titanic rise of interest in mindfulness over the last twenty years can be credited largely to Linehan, who systematized the holistic practice into concrete exercises that could be easily taught to therapists (and, in turn, patients), exported to other therapies, and packaged into self-help books and ultimately smartphone apps. One can now often find Linehan's signature across not only mental health settings but also executive training programs, acting classes, and various corners of the internet. Studies have shown that the mindfulness exercises of DBT—which focus on being present with, and accepting the transience of, thoughts, feelings, and bodily sensations—may be the most effective way that the treatment helps patients learn to regulate emotions and, in turn, improve symptoms associated with BPD.[17]

There is, however, another legacy to Linehan's work that is less positive. Even as some aspects of DBT, such as mindfulness exercises, have by now been branded as helpful to virtually everyone, her treatment simultaneously promoted an image of the borderline as dangerous and insane. Linehan's writing hinted at a deep compassion for those suffering with BPD, but that compassion was often inhibited by the dry language imposed on empirical researchers of her era. DBT therefore had to speak for itself, and its structure largely served to reinforce stereotypes and, arguably, perpetuate the disorder itself.

In strict DBT, patients are seen by group and individual therapists and have permission to call their individual therapist at all hours, with the expectation that the call will be answered. Sections of Linehan's DBT manual, such as "Working out Problems of 'Staff Splitting'" and "Keeping Information Confidential,"[18] were born from the problems that these aspects of her treatment created: patients had a staff to split only because DBT assumes patients need a whole team of people to keep them in check; therapists have a harder time maintaining client privilege when patients can contact them at any time, including when they are not at work, with little regard for professional boundaries.

This was not the direction that treating BPD had been heading previously. Kernberg had seen the condition as something that a properly trained psychotherapist could work with one-on-one, like any other case. But DBT suggested that BPD patients were so wild that only a team of experts, sharing the load and supporting one another, could possibly hope to bring a single one of them back from the brink.

The brink of what, exactly? For Linehan it was something very specific, and the emergence of a new split. Not men or women, passion or reason, good or evil. Not free or confined, neurotic or psychotic. For Linehan, BPD was a matter of life or death.

If you speak with anyone who was trained directly by Linehan, they will invariably define DBT as a treatment for the "chronically suicidal." This was always the language Linehan adopted—she saw the disorder, or the part of the disorder to be treated, in terms of how close the patient was at any given time to killing herself. This posed a problem from the start, as BPD patients frequently engaged in behaviors that *looked* suicidal but did not result in death, and often were not really life-threatening—superficially cutting their skin, say, or taking enough pills to get sick but not nearly enough to be lethal. Epidemiological evidence emerging in the late 1990s and beyond suggested that, despite Linehan's contention that they lived forever on the brink, BPD patients were no more likely to kill themselves than other psychiatric populations, and actually less likely to do so than those with severe depression or schizophrenia.[19]

To account for these issues while still upholding the life-death split, Linehan popularized the term "parasuicidal" to capture patient behaviors that were violent but not deadly. Professionals now call these behaviors "non-suicidal self-injurious behaviors," and colloquially they are often referred to as "self-harm." Contemporary research has consistently shown that there is no clear relationship between suicide and self-harm—some people cut themselves regularly, say, but never attempt suicide; others attempt suicide with no history of self-harm. But Linehan lumped them all together, enough to produce popular concepts of the borderline patient as one prone to make suicidal "gestures," or otherwise threatening bodily harm as a way to garner attention.

In truth, most BPD patients will tell you that, in the moment before they cut themselves, or punched themselves in the face, or drank until they blacked out, they felt consumed by an intolerable emotional energy that cried out for release. They did not want to die, or really to do much of anything other than get the feeling out by any means necessary. Many people with BPD do not engage in explicit self-harm behavior at all—even going by the problematic criteria of the *DSM*, one does not need to have ever self-harmed to qualify for the diagnosis. This is all in line with Linehan's theory of emotional dysregulation being at the core of BPD, and her focus on present, mindful experience—but goes against her portrayal of the borderline as "chronically suicidal."

Linehan, by focusing our attention on the behavioral symptoms of BPD, intended to isolate observable phenomena that could be not only treated but measured. Her landmark 1991 paper, "Cognitive-Behavioral Treatment of Chronically Parasuicidal Borderline Patients," set the stage for DBT's ascendancy and for how BPD would be understood by professionals and the public in the twenty-first century.[20] The paper detailed results from a yearlong RCT in which patients either received Linehan's DBT or "treatment as usual," a common control designation. But given what we know about the state of treating BPD at that point in time—when psychoanalytic advances had been overturned and abandoned, when now-dominant CBT methods had no appreciable success on the condition—it is safe to assume that "treatment as usual" was likely of poor quality. The study bore this out, though the differences between the groups were only cast in behavioral terms: DBT patients were less likely to self-harm, drop out of treatment, or be psychiatrically hospitalized. No significant differences were found between the groups in terms of reported depression, hopelessness, thoughts of suicide, or reasons for living. These measures of emotional change were regarded as less important by Linehan and the cognitive-behavioral establishment that begrudgingly accepted, upon her 1991 paper being published, that her protocol might be worth something.

In prizing the objective over the subjective, Linehan's efforts to define a group of people seeking definition ended up highlighting the group's most extreme behaviors. Even Linehan's discussion of the risks that therapists faced in working with BPD—which Kernberg and others had expressed in terms of how challenging it could be for therapists to tolerate intense and painful emotion—tended to be framed in behavioral terms, measured in patient deaths and the possibility of lawsuits. She developed a way of dealing with borderline behaviors that was both highly structured in its protocols and highly diffuse in its loose boundaries around patient-therapist communication—a dialectic all its own, perhaps not consciously derived but nevertheless stemming from Linehan's own deep and complicated relationship with BPD.

Linehan was born in 1943 to a wealthy family in Tulsa, Oklahoma, the middle of six children. In her memoir, she portrayed her family as extremely mainstream: her oil executive father, a man of "steel-trap integrity"; her beautiful, churchgoing mother; her athletic and socially popular siblings.[21] They were so mainstream as to be, from Linehan's perspective, unequipped to understand Linehan's differences: her physical heaviness in a home where girls should be thin; her verbosity in a home where girls should be seen and not heard. "If a person said something mean to me, my mother's immediate response was to figure out how to change me so they would like me more," Linehan wrote.[22]

Linehan's description of her adolescence is strange and disjointed, indicative of someone who, like Ana and countless others, was severed from her own history, robbed of the meaning that connected one memory to another. Despite being well liked and successful in school, Linehan reported being admitted as an inpatient to the Institute of Living (IOL) in Hartford, Connecticut on April 30, 1961, a week shy of her eighteenth birthday, owing to "increased tension and social withdrawal" and headaches.[23] She was admitted for "two weeks of diagnostic evaluation"—but she would not leave the IOL for the next twenty-five months, reentering free society only at the age of twenty.[24] Though Linehan would not be formally diagnosed with BPD until years later (it was not a formal diagnosis in the early 1960s), her years at IOL marked the start of her experiences as a patient that would profoundly inform her career as a doctor.

Linehan described her admission to the IOL as a "descent into hell," one of many allusions to Christian imagery that also would suffuse her later work.[25] She had been separated from polite society, designated as ill and abnormal, and what followed was not unlike what would befall a nineteenth-century hysteric sent off to bedlam. Linehan was subjected to extreme treatments like solitary confinement and ice baths, cut off from the friends and family who had been a constant part of her life, and exposed to other patients who were similarly disoriented and being similarly abused. It was from these patients that Linehan learned that cutting herself could be a way to relieve an inexpressible inner tension—and to garner special attention from hospital staff.

Though the circumstances come across as objectively horrific, Linehan wrote of her time at IOL with a detachment, at times even a fondness. She explicitly connected some of her experiences to ideas she would later incorporate into DBT—her ice bath treatments inspired the popular DBT technique of instructing the patient to hold ice cubes as a way to replicate the cathartic release of cutting without needing to inflict actual bodily harm.

After leaving the IOL, Linehan's life continued to be a fragmented mix of trying to actualize her intellectual gifts, falling in and out of unbounded relationships with men—especially her therapists and priests, experiences that foreshadowed DBT's unbounded contact between therapists and patients—and looking for a reason to live. She graduated college in 1968 and finished her PhD only a few years later, in 1971, before continuing on to postdoctoral training in suicidology and psychopathology. Even as an established, tenured professor at the University of Washington, where she began working in 1977, Linehan continued to feel plagued by a sense of having not accepted herself. In 1983, she took a break from her university job to stay at a Soto Zen Buddhist monastery in California, where she would learn the concepts of mindfulness that would become integral to DBT. In 1987, she began publishing on DBT theory, shifting to focus on empirical validation studies in the 1990s.

Much of Linehan's personal journey had to be made in secret. She did not publicly disclose her long history of psychological disturbance, nor her BPD diagnosis, until 2011, at a talk she gave at the IOL. Up until then her trip to the monastery and other deviations from the straight-and-narrow professional path had had to be framed to supervisors as choices intended to enhance her career rather than desperate bids to locate herself and stave off a breakdown. Even as she suffered internally, her focus was on how she appeared to others—that is, on her behavior.

"I know what hell *feels* like, but even now I can't find words to describe it," she wrote in her memoir, published in 2020.[26] She was speaking from the vantage of someone in her late seventies, as one of the most revered mental health professionals of her generation. Still, she did not have the words to describe the borderline. Perhaps it is indescribable. Perhaps she spent so much of her life devaluing its description over its behavioral output that she cut herself off from that language forever.

As Linehan prepared to disclose her diagnosis before the IOL in 2011, she understandably worried whether she was doing the right thing, including what impact her disclosure might have on public and professional attitudes toward her work. There is little evidence that Linehan's "coming out" as having BPD negatively affected how DBT is regarded and used. This is fortunate not only in the sense of combating stigma, but because DBT's greatest contributions were informed by Linehan's subjective experiences. If anything, it is regretful that she did not come up in a culture that would have allowed her personal and professional lives to openly commingle, rather than needing to conceal a vast inner world behind the sterility of cognitive-behaviorism and inferential statistics.

DBT could not afford to focus on the subjective—so, it was objectified. This made it great for some patients and ill suited for others. It followed a protocol, it taught skills, it tried to keep everyone's attention on the surface. Linehan's conscientious research, her willingness to play the game of the status quo in which she worked, brought DBT acclaim and made it synonymous with BPD. So much was this the case that people with BPD would come to be told that they *must* seek out DBT, that it was the only choice (as Ana's boyfriend Anders had been told by his cognitive-behavioral therapist). I have also heard of patients being told by therapists that because they were *not* doing DBT, it was impossible for them to have BPD. The *DSM-III* stripped away theory, and DBT stripped away subjective experience—we were left only with behavior and procedure. But what about patients who didn't behave the way DBT said someone with BPD was supposed to behave? What about patients who rejected the procedure?

The mirror was still in pieces. Moving toward the new millennium, people who received the diagnosis of BPD would now unfailingly be referred to Linehan's program—by the same token, those on the borderline who were misdiagnosed with something else would be funneled elsewhere. Some were given drugs they didn't need, or therapies that didn't work, or told that they had multiple personalities living inside them. Linehan had created the largest shard, one that brought specific attention to borderline conditions in a way unseen since the invention of psychoanalysis—but it was still only a shard. DBT took the most visibly extreme cases of BPD and suggested that they *were* the disorder, again severing ties to a more nebulous, pervasive aspect of the human condition: the diffusion of self, the midpoint between madness and rigidity.

11

NORMALITY

Sessions, Year 3

"**D**id you know that Jeffrey Dahmer was diagnosed with BPD?"
Ana asked.

"No."

"I watched a documentary about him last night. It was very interesting. I mean, disturbing and horrifying, yes, but . . . it reminded me that I used to be very into serial killers."

"What do you mean?"

"When I was a teenager, before I was sent off to the program, I'd watch documentaries, read books and articles. I don't know, I was drawn to them. Dahmer said he killed as an act of love. It was a way to possess the person, to keep them from leaving. I can relate to that."

"You can relate to the desire to control another person so completely that they're guaranteed never to abandon you. But you've never murdered anyone."

"Obviously. But I have the same monstrousness in me, don't I? I've gotten in fights, I've punched people in the face. I held a knife to Michael's throat that time."

"It's not the same."

"It's not that different. Sometimes I think you dismiss how crazy I am. You've known me so long now and seen me at my most psychotic, it contaminates your view . . ."

"I would think our history gives me perspective. I've known you across a wide range of states, I can see how far you've come in the past three years. I can see you're not a monster."

"Sometimes I think about quitting this entirely and starting with someone new. Someone who didn't know me when I thought I was dead. They wouldn't see me as someone who's changed, just as someone who is the way I am now. Maybe I'd feel less like a monster with a therapist who never knew I was capable of being one."

"Or someone who didn't know how much a part of you *wished* you were a monster."

"What is *that* supposed to mean?"

"I don't think you were drawn to stories of serial murderers just because they remind you of yourself. It's aspirational. They have something you want."

"Which is?"

"A lack of remorse. They engage in the most extreme of extreme behaviors and don't seem to feel bad about it. What a revelation that must have been to your teenage self, who felt so ashamed all the time."

"I remember feeling like there was something evil in me back then. That feeling intensified during the program, which focused so much on blaming us for our behavior. I've never fully let go of the idea that I'm basically bad and have to fight with intention to be good."

"As opposed to Jeffrey Dahmer, who gave himself to the badness."

"I guess so."

"I don't know who diagnosed him with BPD, but I wouldn't accept that as some objective fact—at least not an especially meaningful one. Being borderline has something to do with that sense of badness, and of not being given the choice to define yourself as anything but good or bad. But it doesn't make you a killer."

"I know that. I'm not saying I *am* Jeffrey Dahmer. But I wonder if I'm *closer* to someone like him than I am to other people."

"What other people?"

"Well . . . this is strange to say out loud. Maybe embarrassing? But I've been thinking about what I want to do with my life."

"Okay."

"I think I want to be a psychologist. Don't say anything. I actually don't think I could take it if you spoke right now. I want to go back and finally get my bachelor's degree, and psychology seems like the thing I'm most interested in. I've spent the last three years devoting myself to this process, but I want to understand it more broadly—like you said, with perspective. I think I'd like to be a psychotherapist one day. But then I wonder if that's even possible. Do people like me do what people like you do? I'm the patient, not the doctor. In a lot of ways that has replaced the idea that I'm bad. I don't really believe that anymore, or at least I understand how it's something I was taught by people who were also traumatized and disturbed. But that means instead of being bad, I'm ill. I know I'm different than I was three years ago. Sometimes I don't recognize myself. I can't believe how I've changed. But I'm also coming to realize that I'll never really be *cured* of this, will I? When you first diagnosed me, I fantasized a lot about how you would cure me, how we would celebrate the day I stopped being borderline. But now . . ."

A silence descended.

"You can speak now, if you want," Ana said.

"Of all the things you could have watched last night, why do you think you chose a documentary about Jeffrey Dahmer?"

"Maybe I was testing myself. I wondered, after all this therapy and hard work, do I still relate to a person like this?"

"Your capacity to empathize with someone other people dismiss as a monster is not an illness," I said.

Ana grew tearful and looked around the room.

"I also wondered if you would think I was copying you or something. I don't just want to do what you do. We're very different people, so I would be a very different psychologist."

"It raises the question of whether you can be influenced by someone without losing yourself. Our work has been important to you, perhaps it has inspired something in you. But you can pursue that inspiration in your own way."

"If I'm being honest, a small part of me hoped that you would tell me that I'm not ready. It's June now, so if I want to sign up for fall classes I'll have to get on top of that soon. But all that anxiety could go away if you think I'm still too sick to take the next step."

I smiled and said nothing.

"Well, shit," Ana said.

. . . .

Date: 8/17
From: Ana
To: Alexander Kriss

Would it be possible to reschedule this week's Thursday session? I was just assigned an undergraduate advisor and I have an appointment with her at 12:30 to talk about class registration. Thanks.

. . . .

Date: 8/17
From: AK
To: Ana

I could meet at 1pm on Wednesday, let me know if that works for you.

. . . .

Date: 8/18
From: Ana
To: AK

That works. Thank you!

. . . .

Date: 8/25
From: Ana
To: AK

I'm still trying to get into a few classes, so my schedule this week is kind of up in the air. The new job is also taking a while to give me consistent hours. I'll definitely be able to make it on Monday; the other sessions are uncertain at this point.

Could you let me know if any alternate times are available? I appreciate it, and I'll keep you posted as I figure out my schedule.

. . . .

Date: 8/25
From: AK
To: Ana

Tomorrow I could see you at 1pm or 2pm. Starting in September, Tuesdays at 8:45am are open regularly if you think that will work for you.

I know there's a lot happening in your schedule right now, but as you get into the rhythm of it we'll be able to work out a new routine.

. . . .

Date: 8/26
From: Ana
To: AK

I don't have a confirmed schedule yet but this week I can do 2pm on Thursday. See you tomorrow.

. . . .

Date 8/26
From: AK
To: Ana

Okay, see you tomorrow at 2pm. Do you want to keep your Wednesday appointment this week in addition, or are we swapping that with Thursday?

. . . .

Date: 8/26
From: Ana
To: AK

I need to swap Wednesday with Thursday. Sorry for the confusion—
there's been a lot to keep track of.

. . . .

Date: 9/1
From: Ana
To: AK

Sorry, can you remind me what time our Tuesday appointment is? I've
mixed up the schedule for the week.

. . . .

Date: 9/2
From: AK
To: Ana

I have you down for 8:45am. See you then.

. . . .

Date: 9/4
From: Ana
To: AK

Hi, can we reschedule our session tomorrow? Let me know what times
you have or call me.

. . . .

Date: 9/4
From: AK
To: Ana

I don't have any other times open tomorrow at the moment. If something
opens up I'll let you know. Otherwise, I'll plan to see you at our scheduled
time on Wednesday.

. . . .

Date: 9/4
From: Ana
To: AK

Why are you dropping me like this?????? You're the worst person
ever. You clearly don't understand how difficult this is for me. I'm in the
bathroom crying and having a panic attack at work because you're
extremely reckless and irresponsible. I have BPD and I've been *relying*
on these painful mind-fucking therapy sessions to help me. You said "we'll
work it out" SO why aren't we doing that?

Seems like "we'll work it out" means I will have to accommodate YOUR
schedule. I hate your hours. I'm not doing 8:45 on Tuesdays. I've only had
5 hours of sleep and I'm already falling behind on schoolwork.

I'm tired of your disregard. I hate you.

Will you respond?

Otherwise I'm cancelling all my sessions next week because I'm not
going to give more of my time to someone who doesn't understand the
fragility of my mental state or reciprocate the same work I've put in for
3 years. Other therapists would. And when I have my own practice I will
hold office hours for the WORKING person's schedule—this is horse shit.
You're a liar. You broke your word and you've left me stranded. I FUCKING
HATE YOU DR KRISS.

. . . .

Date: 9/4
From: AK
To: Ana

I understand that you're upset. I am not dropping you in any way—if
I had been able to accommodate your request to change tomorrow's
appointment time I would have done so. Beyond that, I was not aware
that you were dissatisfied with our planned schedule for the semester
until receiving this email. Taking the Tuesday 8:45am time is entirely your
choice—it seemed the best fit to match both your busy schedule of work
and school and my immediate availability, but if you don't think it will work
for you we can discuss that on Monday. I hope to see you then.

. . . .

Date: 9/5
From: Ana
To: AK

I'm sorry about yesterday—incoherent rage and trapped at work. I knew it wasn't a good idea to send the email. Apologies.

I'm aware that it's my choice so please cancel Tuesday. I'm also unsure about the rest of the week. I really didn't appreciate your scripted, cold response. I don't blame you, especially after the things I said. I'm just tired of it and I'm not going to waste my time explaining what that means for me. If someone needs my appointment time, please feel free to give it away, just let me know. Otherwise I'll try to take the space in my busy schedule to figure out if I can make it on Monday or Thursday or the rest of the semester.

. . . .

Date: 9/8
From: Ana
To: AK

I can't make my Monday and Thursday appointments. Thanks.

. . . .

Date: 9/8
From: AK
To: Ana

I'm sorry to hear that. I understand that you were upset and offended by the fact that I could not see you last Thursday, and perhaps equally so by my response to your email. I replied to you in the way that I did because, as we have discussed in the past, it is incredibly difficult to have a productive conversation about emotionally charged material through email. That remains true now—if you're not interested in talking with me, I'm left with few options to try to address your concerns. Perhaps we could speak by phone sometime this week if you're not currently open to meeting in person? I could speak at 10am or 11:30am tomorrow. Let me know if one of those times works for you, and if you'd like me to block out time for a brief check-in or a full session.

. . . .

Date: 9/8

From: Ana

To: AK

I don't really want to talk but I suppose terminating without speaking to you first would be unwise. 10am and brief works for me.

Thanks.

It is notably difficult for me to recall the phone conversation with Ana. I don't remember where I was or what was discussed. My written note about the call placed it at twenty minutes long but otherwise maintained a level of abstraction. I described Ana as "defensive, combative" and "reflective, at times reluctantly, that her feelings about me might be rooted in longstanding fears of abandonment." At one point during the conversation, according to my note, Ana switched to talking about how she was doing well in her statistics class, which defied a narrative she had been told since childhood, especially by her father, that she was bad at math. "It was as though she suddenly wanted to catch me up on good news, despite her professed desire to cut off our relationship entirely," I wrote.

When I pointed out this discrepancy, Ana acknowledged a sense of inner conflict and said she needed a few days to decide how she wanted to proceed. She said she would reach out to me in the coming days once she'd had a chance to think through her options. My note ended: "Above all, I emphasized my interest in helping Ana make thoughtful decisions that are reasonably in her best interest."

Because this note was part of a patient's official health record, it was not unusual that I kept things vague. In the rare event that I might be compelled to share someone's chart with outside parties—if I were subpoenaed, for instance—I prefer to maintain a chart that is accurate but devoid of unnecessary detail. Nevertheless, I'm familiar enough with my own writing style to look back on phrases like "thoughtful decisions" and "reasonably in her best interest" and detect a prickliness, a latent anger.

I have no trouble recalling that I found the whole situation disorienting. I felt dismayed and hurt that Ana could, in the midst of a transitional period in her life, still see me as a villain and a liar, as she had two years earlier when she'd learned I was having a child. The notion of being a liar, in particular, bothered me. It suggested something active on my part, something beyond Ana's impression that I felt indifferent about her. It was a charge of intentional, deceptive behavior.

Over the weekend, Ana sent me an email that simply read: "Are we meeting Monday?" It seemed a denial of the fact that we had left the matter in her hands. *She* was supposed to let *me* know if we were meeting on Monday. I replied to say that I continued to hold her usual appointments in my calendar, and she wrote back to say she'd be there.

When she arrived on Monday, the tension was palpable. For several minutes she did not speak or make eye contact.

"I don't want to talk about us, but I don't know what else to talk about," she said at last.

"I see," I said.

"A big reason I'm here is because of Michael." They had, by this point, been together for nearly nine months. "I have not been well and he's noticed. It's affecting our relationship. I told him that I hated you and you'd lied to me, and he said, 'Are you sure? That doesn't sound like Dr. Kriss.'" She looked at me and flashed a mischievous smile. "You can imagine how that went over with me. But I realize I can't take everything out on him, and I've been so fucking reliant on you I don't even know where else to go."

"You've been under a lot of stress," I said, which is the kind of placeholder statement I generally try to avoid. I said it to say something, not because I had something to say.

Ana glared at me. "Are you going to apologize?"

I paused, recognizing the need to proceed carefully. "I'm not opposed to the idea," I said. "But at this moment I'm not clear on what you think I need to apologize for."

"For leaving me all alone. For not being there when I needed you. For *lying* to me."

"I know you see it that way. And you're entitled to your anger and your hurt."

"If you don't apologize I'm going to walk out and that will be it, I'm never coming back."

"I won't agree to being someone I'm not just to keep you here. I want to understand, but I won't sign off on your interpretation of reality *before* I understand."

A long pause followed. I wondered if Ana was going to stand up and leave.

"You said we would work it out," she said.

"I believed that when I said it. I still do. But I see now that we had a different understanding of how long it might take. And that I didn't appreciate how hard this transition would be for you. I am sorry for that. Things are clearer in retrospect. We can't experience and reflect at the same time. Given what I knew a month ago—what we both knew—I'm not sure we could have predicted this, or what I might have done differently."

Ana sat with this for what felt like a long time. Then she spoke.

"I *hate* how hard this has been. So much has happened. With school, work, Michael . . . it can be hard to even know what I'm overwhelmed by." She met my eyes briefly and then looked out the window. "On the first day of Intro to Psych, my professor said something like, 'For a long time the study of psychology was influenced by Freud, but now we know his ideas were wrong and his methods were unscientific, so we've moved on.' I was so disappointed. It's not what I was expecting at all, after this time with you. Did you know academic psychologists talk about the mind like it's just a big machine? It makes me so upset . . . too upset, irrationally upset. I've found it impossible to keep myself out of the subject matter.

I hate it—everything comes back to me. Sometimes I sob over my stats homework just thinking about the past. It's *math*, it's the most unemotional thing! At least everyone else seems to see it that way. It's the same thing, the same fucking thing. I don't fit in anywhere."

She looked at me again. Her gaze was intense but no longer seemed possessed by a blinding rage. She seemed to be really seeing me.

"That's what you lied to me about," she said. "You made me believe that I could do this. But it was bullshit. I'm a freak in a world of normal people."

Over the following weeks, Ana resumed attending our sessions regularly. Her anger seemed to have cooled, and she reflected on its intensity: "It felt like trying to contain a volcano," she said of the moments before she'd sent me her most florid email. Yet we never really resolved the question of whether I had wronged Ana in some way by suggesting, in one way or another, that she was fit to participate in society.

Normality became a preoccupation for Ana. She began to talk about normal people in nearly every session. How did they dress? What did they eat? What did they talk about? Sometimes she posed these questions wryly, as though she were an anthropologist studying her peers at college, who were generally several years younger than her.

"There's a lounge area in the main building where I can watch the normies in their natural habitat," she said once.

In these moments, Ana saw herself as equipped with a unique lens acquired by her years of living on the periphery, as well as through the process of coming to know herself in therapy. From this vantage, normal people were naive and untested. The gap she sensed between herself and them could be understood as a function of her having seen things they could not yet understand, or perhaps never would.

Ana's sense of bemused detachment, even superiority, never lasted long—inevitably it would devolve into a visceral feeling of alienation. She did not see her own psychology as existing on a continuum with those around her. She felt she had been knocked off that track a long time ago and now was irrevocably something else, something *different*. Her use of the word "freak" had not been new or incidental—Ana had long identified with this word. She saw herself as inherently drawn toward politics, art, and social groups defined by their place at the fringes of the mainstream. At times, Ana saw her position as a choice, but often it felt like the inevitable result of her being barred admittance to the normal.

Ana's sense of being caught on a borderline between two worlds had dogged her for her whole life. In more traditional settings she'd been rejected as not feminine enough, while in progressive groups she'd been called overly feminine; with white friends she was tokenized as exotic, while with other Mexican Americans she'd been shamed for her limited Spanish. Over the course of our work together, Ana had come to realize that the only glue she'd found to hold many past and present relationships together had been those in which there was a shared experience of chronic and unprocessed trauma. This fostered dynamics that on one hand felt free of judgment but on the other tended to demand that extreme, even abusive behavior be tolerated no matter what. In fits and starts over the past three years, Ana had distanced herself from many of the people who had once occupied so much of her time, as she saw not only that they often treated her poorly, but also that they simply didn't have much in common.

"I used to be sick with lots of friends," she told me. "Now I'm healthier and alone. I'm not sure if I should thank you or blame you."

"Here we are again," I said. "Back to the question of my responsibility over who you feel you've become."

"I didn't change like this by myself. When I think of those early days, I was so lost. I know that I needed someone to help guide me to myself, and overall I'm glad that someone was you. But you and I are *not* the same."

"Who said we were?"

"You have an agenda, is my point. Even if you don't mean to. You have ideas about what's healthy and you've steered me toward them. But they're your ideas, aren't they? Not mine. Like, you always talk about balance between extremes. But what if deep down I *like* extremes and you've led me away from who I really am?"

"I've tried to stay close to your experience—though it's true I cannot separate myself from myself. I certainly have views on extremity at a theoretical level. But I've also witnessed firsthand *your* experience of extremity, and how much pain it's caused you."

"It's still hard, in a way, to tell the difference between inside and outside. Sometimes it feels like you've molded me into a mini-version of yourself, and that's why something doesn't feel right. Then other times it feels like I really am a more authentic version of myself than I've ever been, and the problem is that I've looked to you to help me understand the world, and you misrepresented it."

"In what way?"

"Well, first of all, studying psychology is not at all like I thought it would be. My professor hasn't mentioned Freud or psychoanalysis again since that one snarky comment on the first day. It's all cognitive blah blah and this is how eyeballs work. It's not what I signed up for. And something else happened the other week that really bothered me. I still don't know how to think about it."

"Okay."

"I'm taking this English class to fulfill a requirement. I actually really like the professor; she gives a lot of space for students to talk, but also doesn't pressure anyone to speak. I feel comfortable there. So, I decided to say something about the 'trigger warnings' she had put in the syllabus. I guess they're a common thing, but I'd never seen them before, and seeing them really upset me at the start of the semester."

"Seeing the trigger warnings upset you?"

"Yes. It felt like the message is that, if you've experienced trauma, you'll always be out of control. That you can't do it yourself, you need someone else to decide what you can see or hear, or predict how something will make you feel. I've worked so hard in *here* so that when I go out *there* I can figure out how to exist without becoming overwhelmed. Probably what I said was not very coherent—I still get very anxious when speaking in front of a group. I tried to say how isolating it felt to have these marks on the syllabus, calling out two distinct types of people in the class: the ones who will be triggered and the ones who won't. I tried not to make it personal or get upset. I even related it to the text because we're reading *The Scarlet Letter*."

"I see."

"It did *not* go over well. People got really upset and defensive. At first I was combative and then I shut down. Then the professor kind of shut the whole conversation down. After class a girl came up to me. She was actually very nice. She basically said she understood my point but that it was hard to talk about because there had been protests against trigger warnings on campus last year by a group of alt-right students. I felt like I was going to puke. I said, 'Oh my God, I'm not one of them.' I didn't know how to explain that I'm not one of anyone."

It was early December. Ana flung herself into the office, bereft.

"I'm going to fail Intro to Psych," she said.

"Really?"

"I got a terrible grade on the midterm. She took forever getting them back to us and now I don't know what to do."

Usually, as may be obvious by now, when in session with a patient I choose to follow emotion over facts. If a patient describes something "terrible," I stay close to the terribleness: how it feels, how it might be understood and, perhaps, relieved. But something in Ana's certainty made me feel that I needed more concrete information.

"What did you get on the midterm?"

"A B-plus," she said. She began to cry.

"That's . . . a good grade," I said.

"It's terrible! It means I'm not getting it. I'm not excelling."

"You said you were *failing*."

"I might as well be."

A thought occurred to me. I chewed on it for a moment. It wasn't the kind of thought I often shared with Ana or any of my patients.

"You know . . ." I said. "When I was an undergraduate, I got a B in Intro to Psych."

This is what's known in my field as a "self-disclosure." I offer them only with great caution. Volunteering information about your personal experience brings you, the therapist, firmly into the room and can make a patient feel like their own space has been reduced. It can invite a normative comparison that verges on the invalidating: *I've been through this, too, so you needn't feel the way you do about it.* But it struck me that a normative comparison might be, in that moment, exactly what Ana needed.

"Are you serious?" she said, cracking a smile.

"Yes. It wasn't what I'd thought it would be, either, given my own experiences as a patient in therapy."

Since Ana had grown preoccupied with normality, I'd found myself thinking about it more and more. I started to notice how often other patients talked about being normal. Some seemed concerned with classifying their thoughts and behavior as unremarkable. For others it was quite the opposite—they insisted that ubiquitous experiences like grief and anxiety were theirs alone. I thought about how so many undergraduate psychology programs feature a class called Abnormal Psychology, where students learn about mental illness. As I noted in the first chapter of this book, it was in such a class that I first learned about BPD. The implication was that you cannot be ill and normal at the same time.

And yet, weren't most people exactly that? Wasn't I? Overall, I'd had a happy childhood, a "normal" childhood. Adolescence was a time of angst and confusion, but that's *normal*, isn't it? I was a slight, nerdy teen, uncomfortable in my body and terrified of mediocrity. When I was fourteen, my best friend died suddenly by suicide. I started therapy a year later, and in the meantime learned to project an aloofness that protected me, to some extent, from a sense of vulnerability. Even more it gave the impression that I was no longer interested in having friends—so, for a time, I didn't have many. College was better in some ways, worse in others. I had by then adopted a driving sense of purpose to become a writer and was attending an expensive private university known for producing writers. It looked, from the outside, like I knew what I was doing. Yet from other angles—my friendship with Beth, my frenzied songwriting and performing—I might have appeared utterly lost.

Now I was a psychologist, this weird participant-observer profession that many people regarded with suspicion as a rule. Not only that . . . I was a *weird* psychologist. I identified as psychoanalytic, which was unpopular, but maybe also kind of cool—though I struggled to see myself as one of those cool psychoanalysts. I worked with borderline patients, whom many people also regarded with suspicion as a rule. For much of my life, it increasingly occurred to me, I had in my own way been drawn to the nebulous space between chaos and stability, through a strange combination of having a strong sense of who I am and no idea where I belong.

"Thanks for telling me that," Ana said. "I guess I assumed you were a straight-A student."

"No, it took me a while to figure out what I cared about. So much of this process you're in right now is about finding good fits, rather than feeling like you have to be perfect even when it's *not* a good fit."

"It's all been so overwhelming. I think a lot about what we talked about last year, how there are different kinds of love. I find myself falling in love so easily. I'm doing well in my stats class, which is such a surreal thing . . . I get emotional just looking at these dumb equations because they actually make sense to me. Then I start thinking I should become a statistician, which is just crazy. Everything makes me emotional. I don't know how to keep it contained. The material I'm studying, the professors I like, Michael, you . . ."

"Have you ever wondered why you and I seem to be such a good fit?"

"No. I don't know. I remember when I first wrote to you I liked that you'd gone to The New School. And I thought you had a nice face. Then as time went on you did things I hadn't experienced before. You took my psychosis seriously. You lowered your fee."

"Right, but that's mostly about me. You're a part of this, too."

"I know that. I'm not sure what you want me to say."

"I don't know, either. Maybe there's something unknowable about why a relationship works."

"I thought you believed everything could be understood."

"Have I said that to you before? I'm not sure. You said the other day that we're not the same, which is true. Of course, it's true of everyone. But something binds us. We're not so different. Not so different as you and Jeffrey Dahmer, say."

A lot of things seemed to be happening on Ana's face. She still held the half-smile from when I'd told her about my "B" grade; her eyes were still wet from crying before that. She looked stunned.

"That's a new thought for me," she said.

It was new for me, too. What it meant to live on the borderline had been evolving in my mind for years, and here it seemed to take on a more stable, recognizable shape. As Ana pushed herself to exist in so-called normal spaces like a college classroom, however uncomfortably, it seemed more and more apparent to me how much she *did* belong—not because she fit in, but because she *almost* fit in. Her life experience, her insights, her ways of thinking—that is, her personality—granted access to multiple realms of the human condition at once. This was not an easy path. It had taken a lot of work for Ana to even be able to show up to so-called normal spaces without feeling as though she were being torn apart. But this path was also, it now seemed so clear to me, more than one of illness, or abnormality.

Otto Kernberg had distinguished pathological narcissism from, for lack of a better term, normal narcissism—the latter being something natural, perhaps even beneficial, to our development as individuals and a species. Had no one, over all these thousands of years, suggested there might be a normal borderline?

12

INTEGRATION

1980–2023

I have suggested that trauma is what we call an experience that breaks the rules. The experience can be singular, as with an assault or severe accident; or chronic, as with physical, sexual, or emotional abuse or coercion within an intimate relationship. In both circumstances, trauma invalidates: it forces the person to question what is possible, what is real. Trauma *confuses*. But exactly how things play out can vary depending not only on the nature of the traumatic event, but the internal world of the person experiencing it.

This conceptualization of trauma—which acknowledges objective events but prioritizes one's subjective response to them—is relatively new to psychological theory. The word "trauma" only reentered the mental health vocabulary in 1980, by way of a new diagnosis in the *DSM-III* called post-traumatic stress disorder (PTSD). A formalization of earlier, WWI-era terms like "shell shock" and "war neurosis"—both of which had fallen into obscurity—PTSD was codified in large part because of the numbers of Vietnam veterans who had returned home in a changed state. These men were broken and confused: many had to be hospitalized following bizarre, violent outbursts in which they seemed to believe, despite being in a grocery store or in bed with their wives, that they were actually being attacked by enemy combatants in the jungle. Others fell into dizzying patterns of substance use and social withdrawal. Countless veterans ended up homeless or otherwise living on the fringes of society.

Similar to how gay rights activists and progressive psychiatrists had lobbied to have homosexuality removed from the *DSM-III*, veteran activists and progressive psychiatrists fought to have PTSD included. The extent of the political pressure around this issue was reflected in the fact that the editors of the *DSM-III* permitted PTSD to break one of the manual's central rules. While all other diagnoses had been stripped of etiology, reduced to symptom clusters without theory or cause, PTSD's etiology was embedded in the name: the disorder only existed as a reaction to something that preceded it—stress *after* trauma.

We might say that PTSD finally provided a medical consensus over what to call male hysteria—the erratic, violent, and self-destructive tendencies that had for centuries been glossed over as socially permissible male behavior, especially as compared with the hysterical behavior of women. Our modern era, then, defined trauma as a male experience: as a remarkable event experienced by a man and leading to symptoms that, in a woman, would likely be attributed to something innate. This definition was also gatekept: in order to be granted the only diagnosis in psychiatry's bible that came with a clear etiology (even more, an etiology that implied illness was not the patient's fault), one had to prove that they'd gone through a particular kind of external experience.

The *DSM-III* offered several examples of what constituted trauma, including "military combat," "rape or assault," "floods, earthquakes," "car accidents with serious physical injury," and "bombing, torture, death camps."[1] The list is decidedly militaristic, and the single mention of rape, in fact, represented the fruits of a tireless, yearslong effort led primarily by Ann Wolbert Burgess, a nurse, and Lynda Lytle Holmstrom, a sociology professor, who together had coined the term "rape trauma syndrome" in 1974 in an effort to demonstrate the similarities often observed between rape and combat survivors.[2]

The codification of PTSD in the *DSM-III* opened the door for a new era of trauma research. Two figures in this field, Dutch-born psychiatrist Bessel van der Kolk and American psychologist Judith Herman, would play outsized roles throughout the 1980s and '90s in transforming trauma from its initial, post-Vietnam-era definition into the ubiquitous term it has become in the twenty-first century.[3] Van der Kolk began his career in the 1970s working with Vietnam veterans; these experiences informed his initial view that the word "trauma" should be reserved only for certain extreme events, like those listed in the *DSM-III*, and distinguished from the many things in life that are simply tragic or scary—the loss of a parent, say, or receiving a serious medical diagnosis. He justified this distinction with physical evidence, using new scientific techniques, like physiological monitoring and neurological imaging, that had been unavailable to the few doctors of generations past who had deigned to study traumatic experience. Trauma was more than a bad thing that happened, van der Kolk found: it could be seen in the body and brain—it *did something* to people physically. To van der Kolk, his objective and subjective views worked in harmony: trauma was the event *and* its impact. Only certain events qualified as trauma because those were the events that showed demonstrable, physical changes in those who experienced them.

As van der Kolk and others pursued their research, in collaboration and independently, the confounding problem of the borderline reemerged. Once again, a group of people did not fit neatly into definitions of medical authority, in this case the definition of trauma. Many patients presented with what seemed to be post-traumatic symptoms—often less acute than those diagnosed with PTSD, but still marked by dissociation, confusion, rapid mood shifts, and so on—despite having no reported history of traumatic events as listed in the *DSM-III*. Even their physiological and neurological makeups were similar to those with PTSD: a preponderance of cortisol, often known as the "stress hormone," flooded their bodies; brain scans tracked unusual shifts in their neurological activity as they moved in and out of dissociative states.

The problem could not be ignored for long. Beginning in the late 1980s, van der Kolk and Judith Herman began to write together about the "traumatic antecedents of borderline personality disorder," as they put it in a 1987 book chapter they coauthored.[4] In that chapter and subsequent works, van der Kolk and Herman asked questions that would resurrect some of the earliest days of Sigmund Freud and the dying ones of Sándor Ferenczi (occasionally citing the former and rarely mentioning the latter). Why had no one investigated whether people with BPD, known for their intense relationships with therapists and others, had come from early environments of overwhelming intensity? Was it possible that these patients acted extremely because they had lived through extreme circumstances?

In 1992, Herman published *Trauma and Recovery*, a landmark book that drew explicit connection between the histories of hysteria, combat neuroses, and the post-traumatic reactions observed in survivors of child abuse and domestic violence. She observed the marked overlap between BPD and what at that time was still called multiple personality disorder, and how chronic early trauma seemed to underlie them both. In the years that followed, multiple empirical reports, building off Herman and van der Kolk's conjectures, would be published in scientific journals demonstrating the ubiquity of childhood abuse among those diagnosed with BPD or who showed borderline traits.[5]

Trauma and Recovery represented a push to expand the definition of trauma, speaking for a growing faction within the trauma research community that had come to believe that, in addition to singular events, *chronic exposure* to adverse experiences could be similarly deleterious to a person's physical and psychological health. Herman outlined the insidious dynamics that emerged from early environments that were abusive and from which a child had no reasonable hope of escape. She resurrected Ferenczi's idea of identification with the aggressor as a common survival mechanism that differed from what you might see in a war veteran diagnosed with PTSD, though no less indicative of trauma. In fact, Herman suggested that survivors of chronic childhood abuse might be worse off, at least in terms of feelings of hopelessness, as they lacked the benefit of a pre-traumatic life to which they might expect one day to return.

Herman's broader conceptualization of trauma, combined with van der Kolk's emphasis on how trauma is expressed through the body, catalyzed an explosion in professional and public interest in the subject—trauma moved from a niche clinical interest and talking point of the women's liberation movement to a mainstream term in mass media and across all disciplines connected to mental health. New treatments were developed on the strength of modern trauma research, such as biofeedback, where patients are hooked up to heart-rate monitors or similar equipment and taught how to recognize and regulate acute states of physiological distress; eye movement desensitization and reprocessing (EMDR), a combination of behavioral exposure therapy and eye movement exercises; and therapies centered on Herman's idea of "trauma narratives"—that is, the process of helping patients give language to experiences that had previously defied description. Therapists and researchers also began to experiment with applying existing treatments to their work with trauma patients. DBT variants arose that were focused more exclusively on mindfulness exercises. A new, "relational" form of psychoanalysis—distinct from, though greatly influenced by, the British object relations school—emerged in the late 1980s, resurrecting Ferenczi's idea of a two-person psychology in which reality was seen as something co-constructed in sessions, a joint project between doctor and patient.

Even the psychiatric mainstream had to take notice of trauma's growing prominence in cultural consciousness, creating at times a palpable tension between the need to acknowledge the scientific evidence accrued by modern trauma researchers and an insidious compulsion to deny the realities of abuse in our society. The revised edition of the *DSM-5*, published in 2022, cites "police officers re-peatedly exposed to details of child abuse" as an example of what might precede the onset of PTSD symptoms.[6] It is a nod to Herman's expanded definition of trauma, how something that might not have a traumatic impact in a single instance can, when repeated, fundamen-tally shake a person's equilibrium. But the manual does not list child abuse itself as a form of trauma, even in its criteria for diagnosing PTSD in young children.[7] The abused child, perhaps, grows up to be told she has a disordered personality, while the police officer who filed the report is reassured that his problems come from having had to endure something horrible.

So, what happened? How did a growing appreciation for the effects of early traumatic environments among social scientists give way to the most recent edition of the *DSM*, which makes little mention of such trauma and in fact dissevers its description of BPD from trauma entirely? How is it that the word "trauma" has made its way into popular vernacular—used to describe everything from being overlooked for promotion at work to a bad haircut[8]—while a psychologist under oath in a court of law has sworn that BPD has no relationship to trauma whatsoever?

It has something to do with the rigidity of our current mental health system: the need for categorization, for billable diagnostic codes. It has to do with the bureaucracy of research academia that makes shifting our conceptions—and translating research findings into practice and policy—difficult to the point of apparent impos-sibility. And, I think, it has to do with the fact that change would require restructuring the status quo for the benefit of women and children. For men coming home from Vietnam, the *DSM-III* made an exception to its rigidity. For women labeled as borderline, authority has proven to be far less persuadable.

In *Trauma and Recovery*, Herman proposed a new name to encapsulate the increasingly diverse world of trauma that she and others were investigating, a name that she hoped would speak to both the ubiquity of childhood abuses and the range of ways those abuses could affect a person's development, symptoms, and personality. "The syndrome that follows upon prolonged, repeated trauma needs its own name," she wrote. "I proposed to call it 'complex post-traumatic stress disorder.'"[9] Herman expressed a desire for complex PTSD (C-PTSD) to be viewed less as a categorical designation than as a continuum, one that might unify disparate diagnoses connected through trauma.

While the *DSM-5* declined to list C-PTSD in either its initial 2013 edition or its 2022 revision, the World Health Organization's *International Classification of Diseases*, used heavily outside North America, added the diagnosis to its most recent edition (*ICD-11*). The decision represented an acknowledgment of the label's present value as well as a kind of investment in its future: C-PTSD is used increasingly across clinical settings, and its presence in the *ICD-11* gives the stamp of legitimacy to promote future advocacy and research. It's worth noting that chronic trauma is codified in the *ICD-11* using similar language to the *DSM-5*'s portrayal of singular trauma under PTSD. Examples of the threshold patients need to meet for a C-PTSD diagnosis include "torture, concentration camps, slavery, genocide campaigns and other forms of organized violence, prolonged domestic violence, and repeated childhood sexual or physical abuse."[10]

Herman came closer than most to tying together the loose threads of history that have made the borderline experience so vilified and misunderstood. But she also—along with van der Kolk and others from the school of thought I have called modern trauma theory—inevitably created another split, one that separated the traumatized from the normal. And, in trying to emphasize the devastating impact of chronic trauma, Herman perhaps inadvertently set the bar too high: her case examples from *Trauma and Recovery* that influenced a generation of therapists and researchers were a litany of unthinkable, gruesome deeds, filled with children being beaten with studded belts or subjected to nightly rituals of oral rape.

Of course, it is important that we define trauma precisely and not allow the word to encompass anything that upsets us. But how do we differentiate "the degradation of . . . identity and relational life" caused by trauma from "ordinary personality disorder," an odd turn of phrase from Herman's book that seems to set trauma as the line dividing those who deserve compassion from those who do not?[11] Must we always defend the specialness of our suffering? The tenacity and ubiquity of the borderline experience seems proof that there is no clear boundary—that the line between sanity and madness, health and illness, normality and abnormality is itself diffuse.

Over the last thirty years, trauma has become imbued with a social capital, a desirability. It grants admission to diagnoses that engender sympathy, like PTSD and C-PTSD, and wards off stigmatized labels like "borderline" and "narcissist." It grants the patient the right to suffer, a right that our psychiatric manuals do not implicitly bestow on everyone. At its most harmful, the trauma split has driven therapists or others in positions of power—such as the Californian friend of my former patient Haku—to insist on a singular, extreme reason for why a person is suffering, to the point of blending fantasy and memory or even confusing one for the other. There are many documented cases from the 1990s of what is now referred to as the "recovered memory" movement, in which vulnerable patients were steered by therapists—perhaps well intentioned, but with grossly oversimplified ideas about trauma, derived at least in part from Herman's book—toward believing they had endured horrible abuse in childhood or even infancy that likely never occurred. Unsurprisingly, these patients grew more confused as a result of treatment—at times, to the point of suicide—while mental health professionals and the general public grew more confused about what trauma is and who has the authority to say they are traumatized.

The cachet of trauma hovers like a mist over modern life. It prompts many adults to avoid seeking psychological treatment because, as they see it, they endured no special horrors and so deserve no special help. The more banal invalidations, the chronic denials of selfhood—which exist in a murky space between categories—are devalued and ignored. We need only look to the patients I've discussed in this book to see, once again, that in this shadow-space exists a vast group of people. When Blake's father abandoned him at age six, after which his mother struggled to provide stability, moving constantly, becoming preoccupied with a series of failed romantic relationships to which Blake held a front-row seat—was that traumatic? Rachel's father never struck her, never raped her, never led her to believe her life was literally in danger—so, was the accumulation of his constant insults, his calling her ugly one day and a slut the next, his disparaging any act of independence or creativity she dared to attempt, not traumatic? We run into the same problem that has always beleaguered the borderline, of being defined from the outside in. *You did not experience this kind of event, so you cannot be traumatized.* Because the rest of us cannot see the wound, it must not be there.

Herman envisioned C-PTSD as a continuum, but it has been turned into another category, another mirror shard that further splinters our perception of those suffering from timeless problems. Though Herman openly acknowledged that much of her work in developing the concept of C-PTSD was rooted in treating border-line patients, contemporary empirical research has grown obsessed with differentiating the two groups. Multiple studies from the past ten years have been devoted to this project,[12] caught in a loop of proprietary ownership—that is, a desire to prove that a name is real because it describes something new, a flag planted in land not yet claimed by some other colonizing force. There is, perhaps, also a desire to ward off the taint of the borderline from more palatable labels that portray those who carry them as victims and survivors, rather than witches and hysterics.

In my practice, I define trauma as the experience of profound confusion. I am not a fact-finder; I will never know what "really" happened. It's hard enough to assess my own reality, given how prone we are as human beings to the intermingling influences of fantasies and dreams, how we bring our expectations of one relationship into another, how we constantly feel different things yet always remain the same person. In terms of diagnosis, I prefer the label of BPD to C-PTSD: the former speaks to the patient's experience, not only to what has happened to her. I believe there is value in reclaiming the borderline name over once again severing ourselves from its history.

But perhaps it is time to reject the naming of things once and for all. To at least consider the possibility of leaving the world of categories behind.

Before our story of BPD's history collides, at last, with its present—and before we begin to look toward its future—it is worth stepping back to catch up on the work of John Bowlby.[13] When last we encountered the British psychiatrist and psychoanalyst, Bowlby featured as a minor player in the debates between Anna Freud and Melanie Klein in WWII-era London. In the decades to follow he would pursue his own project of synthesis, attempting to form a new model of human development by combining elements of those two psychoanalytic camps with contemporary advances in evolutionary theory and the nascent field of cognitive psychology. The product of this work, formalized as "attachment theory" in the 1960s, would take decades to gain mainstream acceptance.[14] But in the last twenty years it has risen in stature as a key lens through which to view relationships and mental health, and has proven particularly useful as a middle ground of sorts between the historical tendency to ignore the role of trauma in borderline experience and the modern problem of trauma being used as social capital and diagnostic gatekeeper.

In essence, Bowlby took Anna Freud's interest in reality—how people learn to compromise between the demands of internal and external life—and Melanie Klein's interest in the mental life of infants, and combined them with the works of Austrian zoologist Konrad Lorenz and Scottish cognitive psychologist Kenneth Craik. Lorenz's concept of "imprinting," first published in 1935, suggested that some baby animals—ducklings, most famously—had an innate, evolutionarily derived capacity to attribute the first thing they saw upon being born as their mother.[15] Whether it was the duckling's actual mother, another duck, or even Lorenz himself, the duckling would then follow the imprinted mother, looking to her (or him) for care, safety, and sustenance. In other words, the duckling was born, took in information from the external world, and then *internalized* it, shaping its understanding of the world accordingly. Craik, meanwhile, writing primarily in the 1940s, used mechanistic language to describe how internalization functioned in humans, namely our capacity to create a "small-scale model" of the world in our minds as a means of preparing for unknown realities.[16]

Bowlby's new theory brought these disparate ideas together, arguing that a human infant—among the most fragile creatures of the animal kingdom, born without the ability to move or even lift his own head—possessed an innate drive to seek care from others, and that this survival instinct demanded he internalize the mother, or develop what Bowlby called an "internal working model" (IWM). If the infant was not able to anticipate the mother and develop appropriate strategies to maximize his chances of being fed, protected from danger, and so on, he would die.

By the late 1960s and early '70s, Bowlby's eclectic source materials and ideas had drawn a similarly eclectic group of researchers to the study of attachment theory: disproportionately female, interested in the empirical methods of contemporary psychology while also in one way or another not fully assimilated to the fading psychoanalytic mainstream or the rising cognitive revolution. American-Canadian psychologist Mary Ainsworth was the first to demonstrate that IWMs could be reliably measured, using a procedure known as the "Strange Situation."[17] It worked like this: a one-year-old baby and his parent (most often the mother) came into the lab, a small room filled with toys. After a bit, a stranger entered the room. Then the parent left for a few minutes—referred to as the "separation"—so that it was only baby and stranger in the room. Then the parent returned, referred to as the "reunion." This sequence of events revealed multiple distinct methods of coping and adaptation on the part of the infants, resulting in the delineation of three categories of attachment: "secure," "insecure-avoidant," and "insecure-resistant."

According to attachment theory, it was natural for babies to cry when left by their caregiver—they could not fend for themselves and so would do well to command attention when left in a strange place with a strange person—but once safety had been restored, it was also natural for them to return to a state of curiously exploring the environment. This was precisely how the secure infants behaved: they became distressed during separation but were easily soothed upon reunion, suggesting an IWM of the parent as consistent and reliable. Insecure-avoidant infants acted differently, showing almost no visible distress upon separation with their parents and appearing similarly unimpressed when reunited. The IWMs of these infants were thought to contain expectations of a parent whose attempts to comfort them are overwhelming, often owing to the parent's own anxiety. Such an infant, by withholding his distress, was self-regulating at a precocious age in order to ward off advances that he had come to anticipate as intrusive rather than comforting. By contrast, the infants in the third category, the insecure-resistant, were deeply distressed by the separation and remained inconsolable after reunion. The resistant infant's palpable feelings of anxiety and anger were reflective of IWMs that anticipated an unavailable, aloof, or depressed parent. The exploration that a securely attached infant would undertake once the parent returned had to be forsaken in the interest of ensuring safety—the resistant baby feared that if he stopped crying, the parent would disappear again.

Beginning in the 1990s, British psychologist Peter Fonagy began examining what attachment looked like in adults. He found that by interviewing people about their childhoods, they, like infants, tended to behave in ways that could be categorized as secure or insecure.[18] Secure adults gave balanced appraisals of their early lives accompanied by detailed examples, while insecure adults tended to either give sweeping idealizations or condemnations, or alternately talked about problems from decades ago as though they were still ongoing. Fonagy also found that, if you followed people over the course of their lives, their attachment style in infancy predicted with incredible accuracy their style in adulthood. Our IWMs, it seemed, were quite stable once set in place, and informed not only how we acted as children but also how we talked about our experiences as adults. Most noteworthy of all, Fonagy found that the attachment style of parents strongly predicted the attachment style of their children, suggesting a daisy chain of one inner world influencing another, stretching across generations.

One thing that attachment status did not meaningfully predict was mental illness. To some degree, secure adults seemed more contented than insecure ones, but it was hard for researchers to identify any concrete mental health outcomes that differentiated the groups. Whether secure or insecure, people seemed to establish a way of modeling the world from an early point and stuck with it, more or less making it work for them as they got older.

As we might anticipate at this point, an exception emerged. It had long been acknowledged by those familiar with the Strange Situation that there were some babies who did not fit any of the preexisting categories. It wasn't that they demonstrated an alternative strategy to their secure or insecure counterparts, but rather that they shared a common *lack* of strategy. They acted in bizarre or inconsistent ways that did not seem to hold any adaptive value. During separation, these babies might do things like bang their heads on the wall; on reunion, they might cry out to be held while simultaneously scooting away from the approaching parent. It was American psychologist Mary Main who first proposed a fourth attachment style in 1990, which she referred to as "disorganized" or "disoriented."[19]

Main noted that many parents of disorganized children tended to act unpredictably during the Strange Situation—sometimes threatening, sometimes appearing scared themselves. The infant struggled to form stable expectations in relation to the parent and therefore struggled to develop consistent strategies to elicit the care needed to either foster autonomy or provide a sense of safety.[20] The IWMs of these infants were presumed to be fractured and chaotic, prone to splitting and confusion—a reflection of the environment in which they were formed.

Some studies showed disorganized attachment to be relatively uncommon, while others suggested that as many as 20 percent of infants demonstrated this tendency when under duress.[21] In clinical populations—that is, the infants of parents being treated for psychological disorders in hospitals, clinics, or private practices—the number leapt as high as 80 percent. The fact that disorganized infants had so often been left out of pre-1990 data sets, marked as "unclassifiable," suggested that earlier reports of secure attachment's ubiquity—some studies claimed that up to 65 percent of infants across cultures and geographical locations were securely attached—might have represented an artificial inflation.[22]

Both Main and Fonagy became interested in tracking the disorganized group into adulthood, just as Fonagy had done for the secure and insecure groups. Disorganized infants, they found, tended to grow up into adults who displayed many of the contradictory behaviors of their early days.[23] They might describe a parental relationship as incredibly close in one breath and in the next talk about how that parent was never around. In some cases, these adults would enter into dissociative states during the interview—marked by prolonged silences, incoherent verbalizations, or the onset of a robotic speech cadence—offering observable evidence of the disintegrated IWMs within.

Disorganized—or what, in adults, Main and Fonagy called "unresolved"—attachment was no more a diagnosis than any other attachment style. But mounting evidence showed that infants with disorganized IWMs were at risk for long-term pathological outcomes, including difficulties with emotional regulation, dissociation, and being both perpetrators and victims of domestic violence.[24] It will likely be no surprise that children with disorganized attachments were often found to be the victims of chronic maltreatment, though not necessarily in the grisly vein depicted by trauma researchers like Herman. The path to becoming disorganized appeared complex: some infants being raised in unstable environments seemed more inherently resilient, owing to temperament or other genetic factors, and managed to avoid a disorganized style; in other cases it seemed that a chaotic home environment could be mitigated by the formation of stable, close relationships outside of the home, such as with a grandparent. Without some kind of help, however, an infant's fragmented and inconsistent IWM could create a deterministic loop as she grew older. Such a child was more likely to place herself in chaotic situations and less likely to recognize mistreatment as unacceptable or escapable. This, in turn, made it harder for the child-cum-adult to learn how to self-regulate emotional distress or form stable relationships with others.

Fonagy had been interested in the treatment of borderline conditions since the early 1990s,[25] and beginning in the 2000s he and his colleagues began to draw a line that connected early chaotic environments to BPD by way of a disorganized attachment style.[26] Their perspective can be viewed as an update to the developmental arrest models of the mid-twentieth century proposed by theorists like Michael Balint, D. W. Winnicott, and Heinz Kohut: chaos, abuse, neglect, and invalidation had the potential to disrupt the natural process of development in a child, forcing a recalibration to ensure survival in an unsafe place with unpredictable caregivers.

In particular, Fonagy contended that children who developed disorganized attachments struggled, as they got older, to "mentalize," a term denoting one's ability to think about thinking. Mentalization is the process by which we reflect on our own thoughts, consider what others might be thinking and feeling, and imagine outcomes to social interactions still unfolding. An essential component of mentalization for Fonagy was one's ability to appreciate the *opacity* of the psychological world. We cannot know what others are thinking, or what might happen in the future: we can only hypothesize, and the more we're able to hold multiple hypotheses in mind, the more readily we can engage with others without becoming overwhelmed.

Attachment theory in general, and the concept of mentalization in particular, offered a more flexible perspective on BPD than looking at patients strictly as victims of trauma. First and foremost, it did not require drawing a hard line between what did or did not qualify as trauma: any environment that produced a disorganized internal world was sufficient justification for one's present suffering. This framework also left room for other factors, such as genes and biology, to play a role in how borderline conditions developed in some people without needing to adopt a predominantly hereditary view, like that of Kernberg or Linehan, or a wholly environmental one, like that of Herman or van der Kolk.

Second, viewing a patient's experience in terms of her internal models and capacity to mentalize opened new avenues for treatment. A traumatic experience could not be unexperienced, but perhaps a patient's ability to reflect upon and understand her internalizations could be increased. This placed the borderline experience on a continuum with all human experience. Trauma theory, by contrast, insisted on a binary—a person who had lived through trauma would always look different from a person who had not. Similarly, the lens of biology and genetics held that a person who had some chromosomal or chemical idiosyncrasy would always look different from one who did not. But there was no clear line separating a "good" mentalizer from a "poor" one. We *all* have internal models, templates for how we expect our interactions with other people to go: I do, my patients do, you do. True, a person may begin on one end of the spectrum as a result of early circumstances, but who's to say they couldn't move to another point later on? Illness and health do not live in the past. We can assess them only by how a person thinks, feels, and behaves in the present.

Throughout the 2000s, Fonagy and his colleague Anthony Bateman developed a psychotherapy treatment for BPD called mentalization-based therapy (MBT).[27] Like the attachment theory it comes from, MBT attempts to synthesize psychoanalytic and cognitive perspectives: it acknowledges the unconscious, emotionally driven nature of experience espoused by the former, as well as the latter's embrace of the role that cognition plays in our understanding of the world. Drawing especially from Klein's object relational perspective, which sees human beings as inherently multitudinous, MBT therapists are trained to conceptualize people not in terms of a singular personality but as existing in various "modes."[28]

In one mode, a patient may be freely able to mentalize—that is, flexibly hypothesize mental states while appreciating their inherent unknowability. "He hasn't texted me back," a patient might say. "I'm worried that it means he doesn't like me, but maybe he's just busy. Also, it's only been a few hours, so maybe it has more to do with my expectations." At another point, perhaps even in the same session, the patient might enter a mode that is closed off to mentalization. "He hasn't texted me back and I *know* it's because he hates me." The movement between modes is generally seen as emotionally driven: the more overwhelmed a person feels, the harder it will be to inhabit the balanced mode necessary to mentalize. In recent years, writing on MBT has increasingly described its chief ambition as guiding patients from the "me-mode"—in which they feel trapped with their thoughts and emotions, forced to rely only on internal cues to interpret experience—to the "we-mode," in which their communication with the outside world, including the therapist, can be integrated with their internal cues to draw more three-dimensional conclusions.

Though there is a common thread between MBT and DBT of focusing on emotional regulation, MBT researchers have taken special pains to advocate for their method over DBT. Proponents point to MBT's less demanding structure for patients and the reduced need for multiple therapists or the specialized, skills-based training of therapists. Starting in 2009, MBT has been subjected to multiple randomized controlled trials—doing so was the only way to be seen on the same stage as Linehan's signature method.[29]

Otto Kernberg, notably, followed a similar path at roughly the same time: despite coming from a tradition that had historically resisted empirical research, in the 2000s Kernberg and several of his psychoanalytic colleagues developed—and evaluated via RCT—a "manualized" treatment called transference-focused therapy (TFP), based on ideas dating back to Kernberg's influential midcentury work.[30]

Both MBT and TFP have shown strong evidence as effective treatments for BPD, and in some areas—such as reducing subjective experience of distress—they appear more effective than DBT and demonstrate longer-lasting benefits.[31] Nevertheless, Fonagy and Kernberg have done little to dethrone DBT as the de facto treatment for BPD—it has proven difficult to beat Linehan at her own game. In the United States, it can be hard to find MBT practitioners or ways to be trained as one, as Fonagy and many of the clinicians following his work are based in Britain. TFP trainings tend to be housed within psychoanalytic institutes, which have shrunk dramatically in number over the last half-century and are especially hard to find outside of major metropolitan areas.

I was introduced to the idea of mentalization early in my graduate training—my dissertation advisers, Howard and Miriam Steele, had been students of Fonagy—though I do not practice MBT according to its manualized protocol, or use all of its terminology with patients. There are also many aspects of Kernberg's work, and the traditions he synthesized, that are invaluable to me—though I also don't work from a strictly TFP perspective. I also pull useful elements from DBT, relational psychoanalysis, and other points of view we have encountered, without identifying as a purist from any one group. Humane and effective treatment often requires its own synthesis. Rather than randomly throwing things at the wall, I strive to thoughtfully draw together threads that have long been cut or separated from one another, but can be traced back to common origins.

I do find something especially hopeful about framing health in terms of a concept like mentalization. It opens a pathway for people with BPD to lead less chaotic, more fulfilling lives without suggesting that they must undo or deny who they are. Progress in MBT is marked by increasing one's capacity to reflect—not changing the content of thoughts or feelings, and certainly not the circumstances of the past, but instead expanding the space one has to look at all these things from multiple angles. DBT, similarly, is at its best when serving as a way for people to acquire new methods of dealing with the overwhelming aspects of their inner and outer lives—though this benefit can be undercut by DBT's rigidity and stigmatizing preoccupation with extreme behaviors. Herman's emphasis on building narratives within a trusting therapeutic relationship is essential, but her focus on the lacerating impact of uniquely terrible events has led those who follow her to deny certain realities of human psychology. Herman wrote that recovery from trauma entailed "mourn[ing] the old self that the trauma destroyed" in order to "develop a new self."[32] But we know this is not the case. We always add, never subtract. All the way down to the psychotic core, we can only be ourselves, and the things that happen to us that make us ill also have the potential to serve as sources of empathy and ideas that challenge a toxic status quo.

Mentalization is increasingly being recognized as a concept relevant to people across diagnostic categories, as well as to people who have no diagnoses but nevertheless would like to improve how they manage their emotions or navigate social relationships. In a sense, *all* modern psychotherapies were built on the backs of the borderline, from the earliest origins of Galen's hysterically violent Cretan friend through the invention of psychoanalysis, up through DBT, mentalization, and trauma-focused approaches that are now applied across clinical and community populations. Yet still there is a sense of BPD being something other, less a diagnosis than a curse, undesirable and untreatable. It should be little wonder, then, that some have come to reject the label entirely, while still others have sought to reclaim it, not as a problem but an identity.

In October 2020, a sculpture titled "Medusa with the Head of Perseus" was erected in Lower Manhattan's Civic Center district, surrounded by courthouses and a short walk from City Hall. The installation, a subversion of the ancient Greek myth—which was itself an early depiction of what would come to be called hysteria—was meant to show New York City's solidarity with the #MeToo movement, a global calling out of how men hurt women, how power is abused, and how the oppressed are robbed of a voice and a history. The sculpture was a bold statement in a prominent public space: a beautiful naked woman with hair of snakes, holding the head of the man who, in myth, had been the one to behead her.

Like most anything to do with identity and social justice in the modern era, the reception of "Medusa" was complicated. The sculpture was, for one, created by a man, Luciano Garbati. And, though its sudden appearance in downtown New York suggested otherwise, "Medusa" had not been inspired by the #MeToo movement—Garbati made it in 2008, years before the movement had begun. Who gets to speak for the silenced? Do those in power have a responsibility to lead the way to change, or is their responsibility instead to give those deprived of power, at long last, the room to speak for themselves? Our present grappling with the social order is full of such binary questions, full of contradiction and paradox. Greater appreciation for the suffering of women, children, and racial and gender minorities has coincided with a resurgence in autocratic nationalism, and which way the scales of history will fall remains unclear.

I first heard about "Medusa" from a patient named Eliza. She asked during one of our video sessions—a mode of meeting we had adopted six months earlier at the onset of the COVID-19 pandemic—if I had seen it. I told her I had not.

"It's cool," she said.

"What brought you to Manhattan?" I asked, knowing that, in recent months, Eliza's forays out of her Brooklyn apartment had been few and far between.

"Oh, to see the statue. I wanted to see it up close. I'd read some articles and it sounded interesting. You know, in the photos her face looks cold. She's holding the head in one hand and a sword in the other, and it looks like she's waiting for the next head to chop off. But in person I thought she looked sad. Like she had done something she felt she had to do, but it wasn't what she really wanted."

Eliza's report was most remarkable to me for its specificity. At twenty-five, she was in her second year of therapy with me, and this account was one of the most vivid she had ever brought to session. I could see her standing in Collect Pond Park on a brisk October afternoon, gazing up at the statue. Usually, Eliza's discourse with me was strained through a filter of anonymity—more than anyone I'd worked with, she'd seemed driven to keep herself out of her own therapy. Her words could be a thicket of self-censorship and hedging: "When one happens to feel a certain way around other people, it's like there's nothing to do but leave," she'd said in one of our earliest meetings. Who was "one"? Was it her? And, if so, what was the "certain way" she felt, and why was her emotion framed as matter of passive coincidence? Who were these "other people"? By "leave," did she mean physically exit a space or mentally check out of it? I'd felt further from Eliza in those days in my office than I did later, when the pandemic forced us to meet while miles apart.

As time went on, Eliza became more comfortable using first-person pronouns, and "other people" turned to more precise phrases, like "my friend" or "my parents." But she still demurred on details, insisting that they were irrelevant to a core experience that followed her everywhere: a sense of emptiness, of not really being a person. For brief periods of the day, Eliza felt that she was conscious and perceptive—enjoying a meal, having a conversation with an unnamed friend—but the rest of the time she receded into what she saw as her "default state," which she likened to a computer in sleep mode. She would space out for hours at a time, doing nothing, thinking nothing. Initially she balked at my suggestion that, even if she couldn't consciously access a thought or feeling, she still had them. Eliza almost seemed to pity me for believing there was more to her than met the eye.

Eliza did not meet criteria for a BPD diagnosis according to the *DSM-5*. Her emotions seemed absent rather than out of control, her relationships static rather than erratic. Yet Eliza lived in a profound state of invalidity. She sought to present herself as a generic humanoid, betraying nothing to the outside world: she dressed in neutral, androgenous clothes; she worked remotely out of her apartment, where she lived alone, in a job that required minimal interaction with others; she preferred not to disclose anything about herself to her few friends—even discussing what television shows she was watching felt to Eliza like an act of intolerable vulnerability. But she kept returning to therapy. Eliza said that, though she doubted it was possible, she would like to feel less absent, more real.

My approach to Eliza could not be meaningfully distinguished from how I worked with patients who I more confidently labeled as borderline. As opportunities presented themselves, I pointed out aspects of her experience that she had overlooked—evidence of emotion here, fantasy there—that over time challenged the notion that she lacked internality. Together, we began to construct a new narrative of Eliza's life beyond the simple one with which she'd started: that she was inherently broken and void, a computer with nothing on its hard drive. Eliza recalled a time, several years earlier, when she told her mother she was interested in seeing a therapist. It was after her freshman year of college, and Eliza said she thought she might be depressed.

"She laughed and said, 'What do you have to be depressed about?' Then she got up and kept doing whatever she was doing."

Eliza began to see that she did in fact have an inner world, but that she had cut herself off from it as an act of self-protection: if she didn't know herself, no one could tell her she was wrong about what she thought she knew. She began to consider new facets of her personality: an interest in art, a deep empathy, a fastidiousness. Above all, she began to consider the idea that she *had* a personality, even if she couldn't cleanly fit many of her experiences into preexisting categories, including diagnostic ones like depression or BPD.

Over the last two decades, mounting voices within psychology and psychiatry have called for an alternative to categorical diagnosis. The status quo, as we have seen, has several glaring flaws: two people with divergent symptoms can qualify for the same diagnosis; one person's symptoms can qualify for two or more diagnoses; the presence or absence of a single symptom can determine whether or not someone meets the arbitrary cutoff of being diagnosable. In a nod to the growing dissent, the *DSM-5*'s section on personality disorders included a brief, unassuming new section, titled "Alternate Model for Personality Disorders" (AMPD), which proposed moving away from symptom checklists and binary cutoffs, and toward something more dimensional.[33]

The idea was inspired by the Five Factor Model (FFM), developed by various American psychologists beginning in the 1950s and used prominently since the '90s to assess the personalities of so-called normal people in settings ranging from research labs to job interviews to online quizzes. FFM rates people along dimensions of openness, conscientiousness, extroversion, agreeableness, and neuroticism (often abbreviated with the acronym OCEAN).[34] Could similar ratings of "pathological" traits be used to describe someone's mental illness? Though more cumbersome than ascribing a single diagnosis, talking about someone in terms of their greater or lesser adherence to a constellation of traits would, in theory, eliminate the categorical model's most egregious problems: two people with disparate symptoms wouldn't be crammed into the same category, but would receive a dimensional diagnosis that matched their experience; giving multiple diagnoses would be rendered moot, as the dimensional diagnosis would mitigate any need to try to describe the person across categories; the question of whether someone met an arbitrary threshold for diagnosis would also become irrelevant, as receiving treatment would no longer rely on the patient belonging to any specific category. This latter point, of course, would require not only a philosophical shift in how doctors think about diagnosis but an overhaul of how insurance companies deem that one of their customers deserves to be reimbursed for treatment.

Currently, AMPD is still a work in progress and fundamental issues remain hotly debated.[35] For instance: which traits, exactly, should be used in trying to describe someone with a disordered personality? Should we include the so-called "normal" FFM traits, or confine the model only to "pathological" factors, like one's degree of identity diffusion? How traits ought to be measured is also unclear. If AMPD is to be widely adopted, methods of dimensional assessment—such as questionnaires and structured interviews—need to be developed and empirically validated across diverse populations, all of which takes time and resources. Not to mention the thorniest issue of all: even if researchers and practitioners agree on which traits to measure and how to measure them, how is all that data supposed to be interpreted? If we are smoothing over the cracks between categories, how will we understand a person's struggles and determine what kind of help they might need to overcome them?

In its present iteration within the *DSM-5*, AMPD simply collapses back into a categorical system, replacing its more behavior-oriented symptom clusters with trait clusters. This is an improvement—it is the first time that the proposed criteria for BPD include descriptors of internal experience, such as "anxiousness" and "depressivity"; extreme behaviors are cited as examples of broader traits like "impulsivity" and "risk taking" rather than treated as diagnostics in and of themselves. But AMPD still features elaborate, arbitrary cutoffs—a patient must present four or more of "seven pathological personality traits, at least one of which must be Impulsivity, Risk Taking, or Hostility"—and makes little effort to highlight the inevitable overlap across categories, defeating much of its own purpose.[36]

AMPD is stymied by its adherence to the *DSM*'s atheoretical nature. Describing people's personality traits represents half an idea—we also need a model onto which their descriptions can be mapped. One option advocated by contemporary psychoanalysis is to revive Kernberg's concept of "personality organization," which views all people as existing on a continuum between psychotic, borderline, and neurotic levels of functioning. (The word "neurotic" here encapsulates ways of being that other models might call "normal." The focus is not on separating the ill from the well, but on distinguishing the different ways that people organize themselves.) Personality traits are not just descriptions of thoughts, feelings, and behaviors, but evidence of underlying unconscious dynamics: fantasies, internalizations, defenses against anxiety, cognitive strategies, and methods of emotional regulation.[37]

From this perspective we might synthesize a description of traits—say, someone rated high on dimensions of anxiousness, separation insecurity, emotional lability, and impulsivity—into specific hypotheses about their dominant preoccupations (love, abandonment), emotions (shame, fear), beliefs ("I don't know who I am when I'm alone"), and defenses (splitting, dissociation). There's also no reason we couldn't go beyond Kernberg and also incorporate trauma and attachment theories—models of developmental arrest that suggest people may get "stuck" at certain points on the continuum owing to chronic maltreatment—to give language to the kinds of experiences the person likely lived through (invalidating, unpredictable) and the internal models they may have developed as a result (disorganized, disoriented).

This hypothetical person's personality organization would be distinct from, though still related to, a different person with a borderline organization, whose central struggles might fall more in the domain of narcissism, or a third person operating at a more "neurotic" level but nevertheless struggling with fears of abandonment and self-loathing. Each of these people could be approached as someone with a history and a future; someone who has found a way to structure experience to survive; someone existing in the same realm as all other people; and, therefore, someone deserving of humane and personalized treatment.

We cannot know if what I am describing is a fantasy that might one day be actualized. Moving to a dimensional model of diagnosis would free BPD and its brethren from the shackles of categorization, but it is unclear how, or how much, this would affect the shame and stigma surrounding them. Perhaps replacing the word "disorder" in BPD with "organization" would be superfluous—the word "borderline" is already too laden with the burdens of the past.

Accordingly, feminist and anti-psychiatry theorists have, in recent years, pushed the more radical notion that the term "borderline personality" should be permanently excised. They assert that the label is a tool of oppression in and of itself—a socially constructed denial of the traumas endured by women and their right to have a way of being and coping without being called crazy. There is much truth, as we have seen, in the idea that diagnosis and treatment can be used to marginalize rather than integrate and heal. In one critique from 2005, British poet Clare Shaw and psychologist Gillian Proctor wrote, "The woman is now distressed (and 'difficult') *because* she has BPD, rather than the behaviors associated with BPD being the result of oppression and abuse."[38] They are right. Could BPD or some dimensional equivalent ever be imbued in public consciousness with an understanding of its traumatic origins? Can we flip the myth on its head, or must we reject the old ways in their entirety?

Even under the banner of progressivism, cutting the cord of history can be dangerous. Integrating ideas of systemic oppression into our understanding of the borderline is not the same as replacing one with the other. Boys are not subject to the same cultural bondage as girls, for instance, but the reality remains that some boys *are* denied a chance to develop a sense of self. If we throw out BPD and its related notions wholesale, how will we regard these boys when they grow up? Through the same channels as before, perhaps: we can absolve them through normalization (boys will be boys) or as products of trauma; we can turn them into monsters to be admired, feared, and beheaded. It is harder to hold the middle ground, where empathy coexists with accountability, where a desire for the world to change can coexist with the belief that a single person can change.

Powerful, privileged people and the structures of social life they embody are as capable of having illness as anyone else. We must recognize this, not as a pass for bad behavior, but as a call to a particular kind of action. Much can be done to treat illness, but evil can only be punished. Even if the best we can hope for right now is ordinary unhappiness, the more we see authority as human the less powerful it becomes.

The rise of social media over the last two decades has allowed for a massive experiment in giving power back to the disenfranchised, in letting the undefined define themselves. Perusing the online message board Reddit's thread on BPD, "r/BPD," one finds plenty of terms brought from the world of medical authority—phrases like "radical acceptance" and "splitting" come up frequently, with posters often referring to how they learned about these ideas in therapy. But there is another vocabulary at work on r/BPD that is new and organic, born not from the chosen few of *DSM* committee leaders but the mad egalitarianism of the internet. Someone might write about her "quiet BPD"—a variant not recognized in any psychiatric manual yet frequently cited in podcasts and online articles, denoting someone's tendencies toward social withdrawal and depression when distressed rather than impulsivity and attention-seeking—while another poster explains that he has recently designated a friend or partner as his new "favorite," shorthand for the person in his life who will now become the focus of all his hopes of safety and fears of abandonment.

As a clinician, I am torn on how to interpret the results of this accidental grand social experiment. There is much to be said for homegrown language to describe one's experience from the inside out, eschewing the need for medical jargon that often has roots in condescension, if not outright oppression. It has allowed a degree of compassion to enter the world of the borderline that was hard to detect for much of the last few thousand years: community message boards, websites, and popular social media personalities speak from the perspective of those who know BPD from within, or from the perspective of close friends or family members whose understandings of the borderline are distinct from, but not inferior to, those of doctors or researchers.[39]

But internet culture—perhaps modern culture in general—places a great imperative on self-labeling, of declaring publicly who you are, which can harden the misconception that what we call personality is immovable, immutable, or wholly innate. BPD is often presented online as an identity unto itself, something that *just is*, to be accepted but not necessarily understood. Diagnosis is perverted into a shield against criticism. Invariably, people have invoked a BPD identity in order to justify their abusive actions. In 2017, musician Abby Weems posted on Twitter about the violent and chaotic treatment she endured while romantically involved with Dustin Marshall, a podcast producer, a disclosure that became associated with the broader #MeToo movement. "He made it so easy to rationalize his behavior, telling me 'that's just what happens when someone has BPD,'" Weems wrote. "His personality disorder made up so much of his identity that any abusive behavior fell under the umbrella of his condition. He would say to me 'I warned you' and 'this is what you signed up for' or 'you should have expected this.'"[40]

Eliza, I learned early in our work together, was quite familiar with r/BPD. Though we had never explicitly discussed any diagnosis for her, the internet served as an essential, anonymous way for her to begin understanding herself in conjunction with our therapy. The notion of a "quiet" version of BPD stood out to her in particular, and the posts, articles, and videos she consumed on the subject filled her with simultaneous feelings of belonging and defeat.

"It seems this stuff is pretty fixed," she said. "People don't talk about it as a thing that might get better. Or even something they want to get better. It's the same as what I've always told myself. There's nothing else to me."

The borderline touches all of us. It is *normal*, but that does not make it an identity. In truth, it is the lack of one. It is a place to pass through, not to stay; a waypoint on the path to self-knowledge; an acknowledgment of the universal experience of suffering and the way relationships shape us.

The power to define normal is one of the greatest powers bestowed to any authority figure. Parents set expectations of what children should anticipate from the world; political leaders dictate which social problems are tolerable and which need to be addressed; doctors and therapists decide who is called ill and who is called well. BPD—both its history and the countless who suffer from it today—is living proof of how this power corrupts. Changing this reality cannot only take place in a therapist's office: it requires a broader reconsideration of how we try to push away the realities of human suffering and abuse—how we split, stigmatize, medicalize, do whatever we can to deny the psychosis that binds us, to preserve a rigid sense of normal.

Really, there is no normal. Or, if there is, it's ever-changing and encompasses not only happiness and strength but pain and disintegration. BPD, for its millennia-old status as an outlier, can teach us how to be a healthy kind of normal, if we are willing to listen. It is the story of how one moves from chaos to stability; from a black-and-white worldview to a more complex one; from a life defined by desperation to one defined by a sense of who we are.

13

BORDERLINE

Sessions, Year 6

"We started talking about past relationships," Ana said during a recent session. "I wondered later if it was too much to get into for a first date, but I feel like I can only slow things down so much. I know it's been a problem for me, diving in too quickly, over-disclosing—but I can't stand mindless chatter. I want to talk about real things. I don't think that's pathological."

I thought, *That's why I became a psychotherapist. To skip the mindless chatter and talk about real things.* But I only nodded.

She continued, grinning slightly. "He said that his last girlfriend was borderline. It bothered me, partly the way he said it but mostly just that it was said. It's always there! So, I said, 'Borderline? What's that?'" The grin widened. "Listen, I know what you're thinking. Actually, I *don't* know what you're thinking, but if you're thinking I was testing him, you're only half-right. I'm not sure why I said it. Sitting outside of it all for a second, looking in and saying, 'Hmm, what's that?' . . . I didn't feel like I was lying. I still felt like myself."

"What did he say?"

"Oh, the usual," she laughed. "I don't think I want to see him again. Maybe I do. It's very hard to take things slowly."

"There's a lot of ambiguity."

"Yes. It would have been unbearable in the past."

The past. Ana and I had been working together for over six years. I'd been with her through sexual trauma, unemployment, the return to school and completion of her undergraduate degree, the full arc of a serious romantic relationship, the turbulence of a pandemic that left us meeting mostly online with occasional in-person reunions at my new office outside the city. Each successive event had shaken Ana less, though sometimes that was only apparent in retrospect.

The breakup with Michael, in particular, had tested Ana's nascent faith in a self that existed whether or not anyone else was watching. Over the course of the two years they spent together, Ana and Michael had successfully worked through major conflicts, most of which arose from the fact that the relationship was, for the first time in Ana's life, not all-consuming. The challenge was staying close without getting lost in one another, tumbling into a black hole toward which both of them felt a gravitational pull. In the end, it was this struggle to be together while remaining independent that proved irreconcilable. They cared for each other but wanted different things for themselves.

It was Ana's most profound loss in recent memory. Yet the break wasn't rageful; it didn't happen suddenly; there were no charges of abandonment from either side. Ana felt grief-stricken but not traumatized—losing Michael did not break her sense of reality. Even after it was all over, she believed they had loved one another and felt grateful for their time together.

I'd been with Ana through all of this. But in another sense, I'd been with her through none of it. All we really had together was the practice of sitting in my office—or now, at our respective computers—and talking. Four times a week, then three, now two. So much of Ana could never be contained in a book. The best I could attempt to do was tell the story of our relationship, a conversation over a thousand hours long. Still going, for now. The Ana I looked at on my screen now was, in some ways, unrecognizable to the one who first came to see me. Yet she was also clearly the same Ana—more so, somehow.

"Why are you looking at me like that?" she asked.

"I'm wondering how *you* would answer the question," I said. "Peering in—oh, look, it's borderline personality disorder—what *is* that?"

"I think about that a lot. I don't identify with BPD the way I used to. It's not a commandment anymore, which I guess means you're not God. Sorry!"

"I prefer it this way."

"I knew you'd say something like that." She smiled again. "Okay. What is BPD? It's love and hate, I guess. It's being a person, literally. Does that make sense? Everybody says, 'I love you,' 'I hate you,' 'I don't know who I am,' but most of them don't mean it literally, or know what it feels like to mean it literally. It's living inside a mirror, reflecting everyone around you. It's flat and confined. Sometimes I still feel trapped in that mirror. But I learned how to step outside of it and into the three-dimensional world. Now I spend most of my time here. Don't I? I guess it depends on what's going on. Maybe, like, 70 percent real world, 30 percent mirror? But there's also something I've learned from being borderline. Something important. I don't entirely know what it is yet. A way of seeing things, maybe."

I nodded again. Ana studied my face, deciphering the language written on it that so few learn to read, or even pay attention to.

"Oh God," she said. "Are you going to put that in your book?"

For the third time, I nodded.

Can a relationship change who you are? It is a question that has followed not only BPD's long history but the history of human civilization; if nothing else, it is the question on which my profession hangs.

Early relationships are undeniably important: the people who raise us shape our expectations of the world before we have access to any comparison. My relationship with my parents shaped me: their stability, their love and support; also their shortcomings, the ways they misunderstood me. It doesn't stop there, of course. My relationship with my therapist changed me: he made me aware of feelings for which I'd lacked words, of thoughts I'd wished weren't there; arguably, it set me on the path that would define my professional life. But I might not have seen a therapist when I did if not for parents who supported the idea, believed that change through conversation was possible. I almost certainly wouldn't have started therapy when I did if not for another relationship, the one I'd had with my best friend, whose suicide pushed the problems of my life and personality from the unpleasant into the unbearable.

Relationships are struggles. We want to know and be known, love and be loved. But there is always a limit, a gap. The ways we miss and hurt each other matter as much as the ways we come together. No relationship is linear; therapy doesn't help a person by making them feel good all the time. To the contrary, there is a growing awareness that ruptures in therapy relationships are inevitable—it is neither possible nor helpful to try to avoid them. What matters is how they are repaired.[1] Mending something damaged can, in fact, bring two people closer together, help them see each other and the world in new ways.

Ana is not the only one in our relationship who is different now versus six years ago. I am not the same therapist or the same person. We are part of each other's stories. Still, there is a gap; we still misunderstand each other. We learn new things, the dynamic is always changing. Telling Ana that I was writing this book brought up complicated feelings for both of us. It recalled her father's prophecy that I was using her as some kind of test subject; it made Ana proud of the progress she'd made and the idea that her experience might help others. On days she felt unwell, it made her ashamed—she felt like she owed me perfection; like she'd let me down. It brought to the fore the uneven power dynamic between us. When I asked permission to write about her, was she actually free to say no? Who was I to tell her story?

"I'm not sure if you remember, the time you called me from the subway platform, that day you lost your job," I said once, when Ana asked what I was writing about at the moment.

"Of course I remember," she replied. "Only I wasn't in the subway, I was walking down the street."

"Oh. Are you sure?"

"Yes. I remember it vividly. I was crying and saw my reflection in the window of the consignment shop I used to go to all the time in those days."

This is what makes history, personal and global, so confounding. We can't both be right. Probably, Ana is right. Probably, I pictured her on the subway platform because I knew she would be taking the train to my office after our phone call, and this impression made its way into my notes; a fantasy became a memory.

But it's also true that she *was* on a platform. Maybe not the literal one at Eighty-Sixth Street on which I'd placed her in my mind, but some sort of precipice. When Ana arrived at my office that day, I received her as though she *had* been on that platform—it informed what happened next. This is not Ana's history, it's our history; it's what happens when two subjectivities meet. The borderline, where *I* becomes *we*, where the psychosis of a single human becomes the love and hate, submission and authority, joy and despair that only exist when that person makes contact with another.

One day, my relationship with Ana will end. She used to fantasize about coming to see me when we're both in our eighties, shuffling into my office on a cane, me in a wheelchair.

"Why am I in a wheelchair?"

"Let's not analyze it."

Now she talks about what it would be like to stop. Ending is one of the most important phases of treatment: it is the opportunity to say goodbye, to face a loss that's not an abandonment, as she did with Michael. It's a bridge we've yet to cross. Will I see Ana through future relationships or starting a family? Will I see her through graduate school and becoming a therapist? Ana would be a good one, I think, though there are plenty of other places her creativity, empathy, and keen observations might take her. These questions will be important to Ana's history, but in the history of our relationship they are a distraction. I wonder when I'll let go of my desire to know what will happen next. To trust that our time together, our relationship, has already told me everything I need to know.

"I've started disagreeing with you more lately," she said. "Have you noticed that?"

"Yes. You seem more confident about when a thought of mine is not a thought of yours."

"I have mixed feelings about it—I guess what you'd call 'progress.' I feel further away from you and sometimes I miss the old closeness. Obviously, things were bad when we met. I thought everything started with Tom and what he'd done to me. Now, everything feels less contained, more connected. Tom was just one part of a long story—in a way, so are you."

Change and sadness are flip sides of a coin. Every time we grow, we leave something behind—if nothing else, a version of ourselves. The mounting losses, the weight of history, can feel unbearable. It's so tempting to forget. But, still. We always add, never subtract.

In early March 2020, Ana came into my office and sat down, as she had countless times before. We didn't know it at the time, but it would be one of the last times we'd meet in that office. She kind of floated in, a wistful look on her face.

After a pause, I asked, "What's on your mind?"

"I was on the elevator just now," she said. "I was alone. And suddenly I imagined that next to me was *me*, as a child. A little girl in a cute dress, looking up at me." She swallowed hard. I could see tears welling in her eyes. Those familiar mirrors I'd first looked into all those years ago. "The world hadn't broken her yet. Hadn't made her believe she was broken. I imagined reaching out my hand to her. She took it. And as the doors opened, I said to her, 'Come with me. Come with me. It's going to be all right.'"

ACKNOWLEDGMENTS

Thanks to Tisse Takagi, Catherine Tung, Peter Tallack, Morgan Marty, my parents, my students, The New School alumni network, and the A. A. Brill Library at the New York Psychoanalytic Society & Institute. Thanks to my colleagues and mentors, too numerous to list, who influenced my understanding of the borderline in one way or another over the years.

Special thanks to Dawn Kriss for, well, everything.

My deepest gratitude goes to my patients. What can I say? At last, I am without words. Thank you.

NOTES

INTRODUCTION

1. *Diagnostic and Statistical Manual of Mental Disorders, Fifth Edition, Text Revision* (Washington, DC: American Psychiatric Association, 2022), 754.
2. Transcribed from *Entertainment Tonight*, "Psychologist on Amber Heard's Borderline Personality Disorder," YouTube, April 26, 2022, https://www.youtube.com/watch?v=UF8KlOOSFos.
3. *Psychodynamic Diagnostic Manual*, 2nd ed. *(PDM-2)*, ed. Vittorio Lingiardi and Nancy McWilliams (New York: The Guilford Press, 2017), 19.
4. Irving C. Rosse, "Clinical Evidences of Borderland Insanity," in *Essential Papers on Borderline Disorders*, ed. Michael H. Stone (New York: NYU Press, 1986), 32.

1: PREHISTORY

1. Sigmund Freud, *The Interpretation of Dreams* (New York: Basic Books, 1995), Kindle. The notion of unconscious processes being mistaken for coincidence arises throughout Freud's writings, but it is here that he states most explicitly that dreams, though seemingly random, "are not meaningless, they are not absurd. . . . They are constructed by a highly complicated activity of the mind" (loc. 2418).
2. Euripides, *The Bacchae and Other Plays*, trans. John Davie (New York: Penguin, 2005).

2: SPLITS, HYSTERIA, AND THE INVENTION OF PSYCHOTHERAPY

1. See chapter 8 for the history and theoretical development of this term.
2. Helen King, "Once Upon a Text: Hysteria from Hippocrates," in *Hysteria Beyond Freud*, ed. Sander L. Gilman et al. (Berkeley: University of California Press, 1993), 4–65.
3. Hippocrates, *Collected Works I*, trans. W. H. S. Jones (Cambridge, MA: Harvard University Press, 1868), retrieved from https://daedalus.umkc.edu/hippocrates/HippocratesLoeb1/index.html.
4. Hippocrates, *Collected Works I*.

5. Euripides, *Medea*, trans. Ian Johnston (Nanaimo, British Columbia: Vancouver Island University, 2008), retrieved from https://johnstoniatexts .x10host.com/euripides/medeahtml.html; Homer, *The Odyssey*, trans. A. T. Murray (Cambridge, MA: Harvard University Press, 1919), book 12, lines 153–90, retrieved from https://www.perseus.tufts.edu/hopper; Ovid, *Metamorphoses IV*, trans. Anthony S. Kline (Charlottesville: University of Virginia, 2000), lines 753–803, retrieved from https://ovid.lib .virginia.edu/trans/ovhome.htm.

6. King, "Once Upon a Text," 25.

7. John B. West, "Galen and the Beginnings of Western Physiology," *American Journal of Physiology: Lung, Cellular and Molecular Physiology* 307, no. 2 (2004): 121–28, doi: 10.1152/ajplung.00123.2014. See also Walther Riese, introduction to Galen, *Galen on the Passions and Errors of the Soul*, trans. Paul W. Harkins (Columbus: Ohio State University Press, 1963), retrieved from https://www.stoictherapy.com.

8. Helen King, "Galen and the Widow: Towards a History of Therapeutic Masturbation in Ancient Gynaecology," *EuGeStA: Journal on Gender Studies in Antiquity* 1 (May 2011): 205–35.

9. Galen, *Galen on the Passions and Errors of the Soul*, i.

10. Galen, *Galen on the Passions and Errors of the Soul*, iv.

11. Galen, *Galen on the Passions and Errors of the Soul*.

12. Galen, *Galen on the Passions and Errors of the Soul*, v.

13. Walther Riese, "Interpretation," in Galen, *Galen on the Passions and Errors of the Soul*.

14. Plato, *Timaeus*, trans. Benjamin Jowett (360 BCE), retrieved from http:// classics.mit.edu/Plato/timaeus.html.

15. Hans Kelsen, "Platonic Love," *American Imago* 3, no. 1/2 (1942): 3–110; Nicholas D. Smith, "Plato and Aristotle on the Nature of Women," *Journal of the History of Philosophy* 21, no. 4 (October 1983): 467–78; Dorothea Wender, "Plato: Misogynist, Paedophile, and Feminist," *Arethusa* 6, no. 1 (Spring 1973): 75–90.

16. Galen, *Galen on the Passions and Errors of the Soul*, viii.

17. Galen, *Galen on the Passions and Errors of the Soul*, viii.

18. Helen Ellerbe, *The Dark Side of Christian History* (Windermere, FL: Morningstar & Lark, 1995).

19. Depictions of Aquinas's life are drawn primarily from Jean-Pierre Torrell, *Saint Thomas Aquinas: The Person and His Work* (Washington, DC: Catholic University of America Press, 2005); Renn Dickson Hampden, "The Life of Thomas Aquinas," in *The Encyclopædia Metropolitana* (London: John J. Griffin & Co. and Richard Griffin & Co., 1848); and G. K. Chesterton, *Saint Thomas Aquinas* (Mineola, NY: Dover, 2009).

20. Thomas Aquinas, *Summa Theologiae*, trans. Fathers of the English Dominican Province (1920), Question 92, Objection 1. Retrieved from https://www.newadvent.org/summa.

21. Aristotle, *Politics*, quoted in Smith, "Plato and Aristotle on the Nature of Women," 467.

22. Aquinas, *Summa Theologiae*, Question 117, Reply to Objection 2.

23. Ellerbe, *The Dark Side of Christian History*; Karen Armstrong, *The Gospel According to Woman: Christianity's Creation of the Sex War in the West* (New York: Doubleday, 1986).

24. Barbara Walker, *The Woman's Encyclopedia of Myths and Secrets* (San Francisco: Harper & Row, 1983), 444.

25. Kenneth Dewhurst, *Dr. Thomas Sydenham (1624–1689): His Life and Original Writings* (Berkeley: University of California Press, 1966), provides the most thorough biography of Sydenham as well as the most accurate versions of his written work.

26. Andrew Scull, *Hysteria: The Disturbing History* (New York: Oxford University Press, 2009), 31.

27. G. S. Rousseau, "A Strange Pathology: Hysteria in the Early Modern World, 1500–1800," in *Hysteria Beyond Freud*, 141.

28. Dewhurst, *Dr. Thomas Sydenham*, 46–47.

29. Rousseau, "A Strange Pathology," 183–84.

30. Scull, *Hysteria*, 66.

31. Camilo J. Ruggero et al., "Borderline Personality Disorder and the Misdiagnosis of Bipolar Disorder," *Journal of Psychiatric Research* 44, no. 6 (2010): 405–8, doi: 10.1016/j.jpsychires.2009.09.011.

32. James Cowles Prichard, "A Treatise on Insanity," in *Essential Papers on Borderline Disorders*, ed. Michael H. Stone (New York: New York University Press, 1986), 14.

33. Irving C. Rosse, "Clinical Evidences of Borderland Insanity," in *Essential Papers on Borderline Disorders*, ed. Michael H. Stone (New York: NYU Press, 1986).

34. My depiction of Charcot's demonstration is not based on a verbatim transcript. It is drawn from general descriptions found in George Makari, *Revolution in Mind: The Creation of Psychoanalysis* (New York: HarperCollins, 2008), and Charcot's write-ups of non-hysteria case presentations found in Jean-Martin Charcot, *Charcot the Clinician: The Tuesday Lessons*, trans. Christopher G. Goetz (New York: Raven Press, 1987).

35. The most thorough cataloguing of Freud's pre-psychoanalytic professional life can be found in Joel Whitebook, *Freud: An Intellectual Biography* (Cambridge, MA: Cambridge University Press, 2017). Freud's pursuit of "the eel question" is detailed in Patrik Svensson, *The Book of Eels: Our Enduring Fascination with the Most Mysterious Creature in the Natural World* (New York: Ecco, 2020).

3: PSYCHIC DEATH

1. Freud introduced the concept of repetition compulsion in a 1914 essay and later expanded upon it in a 1920 essay: Sigmund Freud, "Remembering, Repeating, and Working Through," in *The Penguin Freud Reader* (New York: Penguin, 2006), 391–401; Sigmund Freud, "Beyond the Pleasure Principle," in *The Penguin Freud Reader*, 132–95.

2. Anthony Stevens, *Jung: A Brief Insight* (New York: Sterling, 2011); Timothy Leary, *Exo-Psychology: A Manual on the Use of the Human Nervous System According to the Instructions of the Manufacturers* (London: Forgotten Books, 2018).

3. Freud, "Beyond the Pleasure Principle."

4. Slavoj Žižek, "Are We Allowed to Enjoy Daphnée du Maurier?," Lacan. com, 2004, https://www.lacan.com/zizdaphmaur.htm.

5. Chris Good, "Picture of the Day: Mitt Romney's Money Shot," *The Atlantic*, October 13, 2011, https://www.theatlantic.com/politics/archive /2011/10/picture-of-the-day-mitt-romneys-money-shot/246658.

4: SEDUCTION AND FANTASY

1. Sigmund Freud, "The Aetiology of Hysteria," in *The Standard Edition of the Complete Psychological Works of Sigmund Freud*, vol. 3, trans. James Strachey (London: Hogarth Press, 1955), 192.

2. H. Dubovsky, "The Jewish Contribution to Medicine, Part II: The 19th and 20th Centuries," *South African Medical Journal* 76, no. 2 (1989): 67–70.

3. Edward Shorter, "Women and Jews in a Private Nervous Clinic in Late Nineteenth-Century Vienna," *Medical History* 33, no. 2 (1989): 149–83, doi: 10.1017/S002572730004922X.

4. *The Complete Letters of Sigmund Freud to Wilhelm Fliess, 1887–1904*, trans. and ed. Jeffrey Moussaieff Masson (Cambridge, MA: Belknap Press, 1985), 184.

5. Sigmund Freud, *Three Essays on the Theory of Sexuality*, trans. James Strachey (New York: Basic Books, 1975); Sigmund Freud, *Civilization and Its Discontents*, trans. David McLintock (New York: Penguin, 2004).

6. Freud, "The Aetiology of Hysteria," 197.

7. Freud, "The Aetiology of Hysteria," 212.

8. Josef Breuer and Sigmund Freud, "Studies on Hysteria," in *The Standard Edition of the Complete Psychological Works of Sigmund Freud*, vol. 2, trans. James Strachey (London: Hogarth Press, 1955).

9. Breuer and Freud, "Studies on Hysteria," 305. Freud's radical pessimism has been the subject of much scholarly discussion, though its implications—and the ways it has been denied and "forgotten" by modern psychiatry and psychology—are most vividly explored in Russell Jacoby, *Social Amnesia: A Critique of Contemporary Psychology* (London: Routledge, 2017).

10. Freud, "The Aetiology of Hysteria," 217.

11. *The Complete Letters of Sigmund Freud to Wilhelm Fliess*, 184.

12. Peter Gay, *Freud: A Life for Our Time* (New York: W. W. Norton, 1988), xv.

13. I primarily relied on four biographies of Freud to represent the reverent-critical continuum: Ernest Jones, *The Life and Work of Sigmund Freud*, vols. 1–3 (New York: Basic Books, 1957), the most idolizing and censored of the lot, though also the oldest and the only one written by

someone who knew Freud personally; Peter Gay, *Freud*, an exhaustive and acclaimed work that nevertheless distorts, at times, through the lens of blind reverence; and two more recent texts that incorporate newer findings about Freud's life as well as critical perspectives on his work from feminist psychoanalysis and other schools of thought, Adam Philips, *Becoming Freud: The Making of a Psychoanalyst* (New Haven, CT: Yale University Press, 2014), and Joel Whitebook, *Freud: An Intellectual Biography* (Cambridge, MA: Cambridge University Press, 2017). George Makari, *Revolution in Mind: The Creation of Psychoanalysis* (New York: HarperCollins, 2008), and Walter A. Stewart, *Psychoanalysis: The First Ten Years, 1888–1898* (New York: Macmillan, 1967), also provided invaluable information and context.

14. *The Complete Letters of Sigmund Freud to Wilhelm Fliess*, 264.
15. Freud, *Three Essays on the Theory of Sexuality*, 31.
16. Sigmund Freud, *An Autobiographical Study*, trans. James Strachey (New York: W. W. Norton, 1989); Sigmund Freud, *The Psychopathology of Everyday Life* (New York: Macmillan, 1916), 55–68; and *The Complete Letters of Sigmund Freud to Wilhelm Fliess*, 269.
17. Sigmund Freud, *The Interpretation of Dreams* (New York: Basic Books, 1995), Kindle, loc. 347.
18. *The Complete Letters of Sigmund Freud to Wilhelm Fliess*, 264.
19. Sigmund Freud, *A Case of Hysteria (Dora)*, trans. Anthea Bell (Oxford: Oxford University Press, 2013), 24. Bell's translation of the Dora study is my favorite by some distance, and this edition also benefits from an excellent introductory essay by Ritchie Robertson.
20. Freud, *A Case of Hysteria*, 21.
21. Freud, *A Case of Hysteria*, 21.
22. Freud, *A Case of Hysteria*, 93.
23. Freud, *A Case of Hysteria*.
24. The concept of "false memories" is discussed in chapter 12.

5: FEARS

1. Wilfred R. Bion, *A Memoir of the Future* (New York: Routledge, 1991), 38.

6: CONFUSION OF THE TONGUES

1. Sigmund Freud, "Observations on Transference-Love (Further Recommendations on the Technique of Psycho-Analysis III)," in *The Standard Edition of the Complete Psychological Works of Sigmund Freud*, vol. 12 (London: Hogarth Press, 1995), 160–61.
2. My analysis of Ferenczi relies primarily on George Makari, *Revolution in Mind: The Creation of Psychoanalysis* (New York: HarperCollins, 2008); Ernst Falzeder and Eva Brabant, eds., *The Correspondence of Sigmund Freud and Sándor Ferenczi*, vols. 1–3, trans. P. T. Hoffer (Cambridge, MA: The Belknap Press of Harvard University Press, 1993–2000); *Ferenczi's Influence on Contemporary Psychoanalytic Traditions*, ed. Aleksandar Dimitrijević et al. (New York: Routledge, 2018); and Sándor

Ferenczi, *The Clinical Diary of Sándor Ferenczi*, ed. Judith Dupont, trans. Michael Balint and Nicola Zarday Jackson (Cambridge, MA: Harvard University Press, 1995).

3. Ferenczi, *The Clinical Diary of Sándor Ferenczi*, 99.
4. Makari, *Revolution in Mind*, 272.
5. Emanuel Berman, "A Fateful Quadrangle: Sándor Ferenczi, Sigmund Freud, Gizella Palos-Ferenczi, and Elma Palos-Laurvik," in *Ferenczi's Influence on Contemporary Psychoanalytic Traditions*, 41.
6. Berman, "A Fateful Quadrangle."
7. Berman, "A Fateful Quadrangle," 46.
8. Berman, "A Fateful Quadrangle," 41.
9. Berman, "A Fateful Quadrangle."
10. Berman, "A Fateful Quadrangle," 42.
11. Berman, "A Fateful Quadrangle," 43.
12. Carlo Bonomi, "Ferenczi's Analyses with Freud," in *Ferenczi's Influence on Contemporary Psychoanalytic Traditions*, 35.
13. Berman, "A Fateful Quadrangle," 46.
14. I first encountered the connection between male hysteria and the "war neuroses" of World War I in Juliet Mitchell, *Mad Men and Medusas: Reclaiming Hysteria* (New York: Basic Books, 2000). That book, along with Mitchell's *Psychoanalysis and Feminism: A Radical Reassessment of Freudian Psychoanalysis* (New York: Basic Books, 2000), significantly informs my perspective on psychoanalysis in general and hysterical phenomena in particular. Earlier sources, such as Alan Krohn, *Hysteria: The Elusive Neurosis* (New York: International Universities Press, 1978)—see chapter 8—also drew a historical line between male hysteria and combat stress, though that line was never widely accepted by mainstream psychiatry.
15. Andrew Scull, *Hysteria: The Disturbing History* (New York: Oxford University Press, 2009), 153.
16. Sigmund Freud, "Beyond the Pleasure Principle," in *The Penguin Freud Reader* (New York: Penguin, 2006), 139.
17. Andreas Hamburger, "Ferenczi's Work on War Neurosis and Its Historical Context," in *Ferenczi's Influence on Contemporary Psychoanalytic Traditions*, 65.
18. Ferenczi, *The Clinical Diary of Sándor Ferenczi*, xiii.
19. Ferenczi, *The Clinical Diary of Sándor Ferenczi*, 40.
20. Krisztián Kapusi, "Amidst Hills, Creeks and Books: Sándor Ferenczi's Childhood in Miskolc," in *Ferenczi's Influence on Contemporary Psychoanalytic Traditions*, 8.
21. Ferenczi, *The Clinical Diary of Sándor Ferenczi*, xii.
22. Ferenczi, *The Clinical Diary of Sándor Ferenczi*, xiii.
23. Ferenczi, *The Clinical Diary of Sándor Ferenczi*, 184–85.
24. Sándor Ferenczi, "Confusion of the Tongues Between the Adults and the Child—(The Language of Tenderness and of Passion)," *International Journal of Psycho-Analysis* 30 (1949): 225–30.

25. Ferenczi, "Confusion of the Tongues Between the Adults and the Child."
26. Ferenczi, "Confusion of the Tongues Between the Adults and the Child."
27. Ernest Jones, *The Life and Work of Sigmund Freud*, vols. 1–3 (New York: Basic Books, 1957), 176.

7: LOVE

1. Gabriele Cassullo, "Ferenczi Before Freud," in *Ferenczi's Influence on Contemporary Psychoanalytic Traditions*, ed. Aleksandar Dimitrijević et al. (New York: Routledge, 2018) 21.
2. Lawrence Friedman, "Is There a Special Psychoanalytic Love?," *Journal of the American Psychoanalytic Association* 53 (2005): 351. See also Steven J. Ellman, "Analytic Trust and Transference: Love, Healing Ruptures and Facilitating Repairs," *Psychoanalytic Inquiry* 27 (2007): 246–63.
3. Friedman, "Is There a Special Psychoanalytic Love?," 357–64.
4. Friedman, "Is There a Special Psychoanalytic Love?," 363.

8: IDENTITY CRISES

1. Peter Gay, *Freud: A Life for Our Time* (New York: W. W. Norton, 1988), 434.
2. Biographical analysis of Klein comes primarily from Meira Likierman, *Melanie Klein: Her Work in Context* (London: Continuum, 2001); George Makari, *Revolution in Mind: The Creation of Psychoanalysis* (New York: HarperCollins, 2008); and the Melanie Klein Trust, https://melanie-klein-trust.org.uk.
3. Joseph Aguayo, "Historicising the Origins of Kleinian Psychoanalysis," *International Journal of Psychoanalysis* 78 (1997): 1168.
4. Melanie Klein, "The Development of a Child," in *The Collected Works of Melanie Klein*, vol. 1 (London: Karnac, 2017), 42.
5. Klein, "The Development of a Child," 41.
6. No book helped me understand Klein's wild and essential ideas more than Thomas Ogden, *The Matrix of the Mind: Object Relations and the Psychoanalytic Dialogue* (London: Karnac, 1990). See also Melanie Klein, *Envy and Gratitude and Other Works 1946–1963* (New York: Free Press, 1975).
7. Melanie Klein, "The Importance of Symbol Formation in the Development of the Ego," in *The Selected Melanie Klein*, ed. Juliet Mitchell (New York: Free Press, 1986), 96.
8. Sigmund Freud, "The Ego and the Id," in *The Standard Edition of the Complete Psychological Works of Sigmund Freud*, vol. 19, *The Ego and the Id and Other Works* (London: Hogarth Press, 1964), 1–66.
9. W. R. D. Fairbairn, *Psychoanalytic Studies of the Personality* (New York: Routledge, 1994).
10. Michael Balint, *The Basic Fault: Therapeutic Aspects of Regression* (1968; repr., Evanston, IL: Northwestern University Press, 1992), 19.
11. Balint, *The Basic Fault*, 22.
12. Adolph Stern, "Psychoanalytic Investigation of and Therapy in the Border Line Group of Neuroses," in *Essential Papers on Borderline*

Disorders, ed. Michael H. Stone (New York: New York University Press, 1986), 54.

13. Christopher Turner, "Adventures in the Orgasmatron," *New York Times*, September 23, 2011, https://www.nytimes.com/2011/09/23/books/review/adventures-in-the-orgasmatron.html.

14. Turner, "Adventures in the Orgasmatron," 109–21.

15. Andrew Scull, *Hysteria: The Disturbing History* (New York: Oxford University Press, 2009), 174–89.

16. Office of the Surgeon General, Army Service Forces, "Nomenclature of Psychiatric Disorders and Reactions: War Department Technical Bulletin, Medical 203," *Journal of Clinical Psychology* 2 (1946): 289–96. Reprinted in *Journal of Clinical Psychology* 56, no. 7 (2000): 925–34.

17. Turner, "Adventures in the Orgasmatron."

18. Historical context regarding the creation of the first three editions of the *DSM* comes from Allan V. Horwitz, *DSM: A History of Psychiatry's Bible* (Baltimore: Johns Hopkins University Press, 2021); Edward Shorter, "The History of Nosology and the Rise of the Diagnostic and Statistical Manual of Mental Disorders," *Dialogues in Clinical Neuroscience* 17, no. 1 (2015): 59–67; Rick Mayes and Allan V. Horwitz, "DSM-III and the Revolution in the Classification of Mental Illness," *Journal of the History of the Behavioral Sciences* 41, no. 3 (2005): 249–67, doi: 10.1002/jhbs.20103; and Michael Strand, "Where Do Classifications Come From? The DSM-III, the Transformation of American Psychiatry, and the Problem of Origins in the Sociology of Knowledge," *Theory and Society* 40, no. 3 (2011): 273–313, doi: 10.1007/s11186-011-9142-8.

19. *Diagnostic and Statistical Manual of Mental Disorders* (Washington, DC: American Psychiatric Association, 1952), 12.

20. *Diagnostic and Statistical Manual of Mental Disorders*, 35.

21. *Diagnostic and Statistical Manual of Mental Disorders*, 35–36.

22. *Diagnostic and Statistical Manual of Mental Disorders*, 37.

23. *Diagnostic and Statistical Manual of Mental Disorders*, 38–39.

24. *Diagnostic and Statistical Manual of Mental Disorders*, 40–42.

25. David Rapaport et al., *Diagnostic Psychological Testing* (New York: International Universities Press, 1968), 57–58.

26. Helene Deutsch, "Some Forms of Emotional Disturbance and Their Relationship to Schizophrenia," in Stone, *Essential Papers on Borderline Disorders*, 74–91.

27. Alan Krohn, *Hysteria: The Elusive Neurosis* (New York: International Universities Press, 1978), 194.

28. Krohn, *Hysteria*, 196.

29. David Shapiro, *Neurotic Styles* (New York: Basic Books, 1999), 169–75; John Frosch, "The Psychotic Character: Clinical Psychiatric Considerations," in Stone, *Essential Papers on Borderline Disorders*, 263–78.

30. Robert P. Knight, "Borderline States," in Stone, *Essential Papers on Borderline Disorders*, 161.

31. Otto Kernberg, *Borderline Conditions and Pathological Narcissism* (New York: Jason Aronson, 1975), 3.

32. Kernberg, *Borderline Conditions and Pathological Narcissism*, 41.

33. Ali Amad et al., "Genetics of Borderline Personality Disorder: Systematic Review and Proposal of an Integrative Model," *Neuroscience and Biobehavioral Reviews* 40 (2014): 6–19, doi: 10.1016/j.neubiorev.2014 .01.003.

34. Kernberg, *Borderline Conditions and Pathological Narcissism*, 315–43.

35. Kernberg, *Borderline Conditions and Pathological Narcissism*, 234.

36. Heinz Kohut, *The Restoration of the Self* (Chicago: University of Chicago Press, 2009), 183–91.

37. Kohut, *The Restoration of the Self*, 192–93.

38. *Diagnostic and Statistical Manual of Mental Disorders*, 3rd ed. (Washington, DC: American Psychiatric Association, 1980), 322.

39. *DSM-III*, 322–23.

40. *DSM-III*, 315.

41. *DSM-III*, 317.

42. *Diagnostic and Statistical Manual of Mental Disorders*, 5th ed. (Washington, DC: American Psychiatric Association, 2013), 671 and 666, respectively.

10: DIFFUSION

1. Mark Miller, "Unmasking Sybil," *Newsweek*, January 24, 1999, https:// www.newsweek.com/unmasking-sybil-165174.

2. Richard P. Kluft, "Cornelia B. Wilbur, M.D.," *Dissociation* 5, no. 2 (1992): 71–72.

3. Debbie Nathan, *Sybil Exposed: The Extraordinary Story Behind the Famous Multiple Personality Case* (New York: Free Press, 2011), 209–21.

4. *Diagnostic and Statistical Manual of Mental Disorders*, 3rd ed. (Washington, DC: American Psychiatric Association, 1980), 257–59; Cornelia B. Wilbur, "Treatment of Multiple Personality," *Psychiatric Annals* 14, no. 1 (1984): 27–33. Wilbur considered her most important contribution to the field to be a paper titled "Transference in Multiple Personalities," which she presented to the American Academy of Psychoanalysis in 1959 but did not appear anywhere in print until 1988, in the journal *Dissociation*.

5. *Diagnostic and Statistical Manual of Mental Disorders*, 4th ed. (Washington, DC: American Psychiatric Association, 1994), 484–87.

6. Retro Report, "Is Multiple Personality Disorder Real? One Woman's Story," YouTube, February 24, 2017, https://www.youtube.com/watch?v =STWoc9N3nl8.

7. Camilo J. Ruggero et al., "Borderline Personality Disorder and the Misdiagnosis of Bipolar Disorder," *Journal of Psychiatric Research* 44, no. 6 (2010): 405–8, doi: 10.1016/j.jpsychires.2009.09.011.

8. *DSM-III*, 218–20.

9. Albert Ellis and Catharine MacLaren, *Rational Emotive Behavior Therapy: A Therapist's Guide* (Oakland, CA: Impact, 1998).

10. Judith S. Beck, *Cognitive Behavior Therapy: Basics and Beyond* (New York: Taylor & Francis, 2011).

11. Allan V. Horwitz, *DSM: A History of Psychiatry's Bible* (Baltimore: Johns Hopkins University Press, 2021), 76.

12. Marsha M. Linehan, *Cognitive-Behavioral Treatment of Borderline Personality Disorder* (New York: The Guilford Press, 1993), 35.

13. Linehan, *Cognitive-Behavioral Treatment of Borderline Personality Disorder*, 202–4.

14. Marsha M. Linehan, *Building a Life Worth Living: A Memoir* (New York: Random House, 2021), 304.

15. Charles R. Swenson, "How Can We Account for DBT's Widespread Popularity?," *Clinical Psychology: Science and Practice* 7, no. 1 (2000): 87–91.

16. Thích Nhất Hạnh, *The Miracle of Mindfulness* (1975; repr., Boston: Beacon Press, 1999).

17. Stacy Shaw Welch et al., "Mindfulness in Dialectical Behavior Therapy (DBT) for Borderline Personality Disorder," in *Mindfulness-Based Treatment Approaches: Clinician's Guide to Evidence Base and Applications*, ed. Ruth A. Baer (Burlington, MA: Academic Press, 2006), 117–38.

18. Linehan, *Cognitive-Behavioral Treatment of Borderline Personality Disorder*, 431 and 434, respectively.

19. J. M. Bertolote et al., "Psychiatric Diagnoses and Suicide: Revisiting the Evidence," *Crisis: The Journal of Crisis Intervention and Suicide Prevention* 25, no. 4 (2004): 147–55.

20. Marsha M. Linehan et al., "Cognitive-Behavioral Treatment of Chronically Parasuicidal Borderline Patients," *Archives of General Psychiatry* 48 (1991): 1060–64.

21. Linehan, *Building a Life Worth Living*, 13.

22. Linehan, *Building a Life Worth Living*, 16–17.

23. Linehan, *Building a Life Worth Living*, 18.

24. Linehan, *Building a Life Worth Living*, 19.

25. Linehan, *Building a Life Worth Living*, 18.

26. Linehan, *Building a Life Worth Living*, 23.

12: INTEGRATION

1. *Diagnostic and Statistical Manual of Mental Disorders*, 3rd ed. (Washington, DC: American Psychiatric Association, 1980), 236.

2. Ann W. Burgess and Lynda L. Holmstrom, "Rape Trauma Syndrome," *American Journal of Psychiatry* 131, no. 9 (1974): 981–86, doi: 10.1176/ajp.131.9.981.

3. In addition to works cited later, my depiction of van der Kolk's work and influence comes chiefly from Bessel van der Kolk, *The Body Keeps the Score: Brain, Mind, and Body in the Healing of Trauma* (New York: Penguin, 2015).

4. Judith L. Herman and Bessel A. van der Kolk, "Traumatic Antecedents of Borderline Personality Disorder," in *Psychological Trauma*, ed. Bessel van der Kolk (Washington, DC: American Psychiatric Association, 1987), 111–26. See also Bessel A. van der Kolk et al., "Trauma and the Development of Borderline Personality Disorder," *Psychiatric Clinics of North America* 17, no. 4 (1994): 715–30, doi: 10.1016/S0193-953X(18)30082-0.
5. Lee H. Schwecke, "Childhood Sexual Abuse, PTSD, and Borderline Personality Disorder," *Journal of Psychosocial Nursing and Mental Health Services* 47, no. 7 (2009): 4–6, doi: 10.3928/02793695-20090527-05.
6. *Diagnostic and Statistical Manual of Mental Disorders, Fifth Edition, Text Revision* (Washington, DC: American Psychiatric Association, 2022), 271.
7. *DSM-5*, 272.
8. Sarah Bahr, "'Emily in Paris' Star Lily Collins on Her Own Trauma Haircut," *New York Times*, December 21, 2022, https://www.nytimes.com/2022/12/21/style/emily-in-paris-cast-lily-collins.html.
9. Judith Lewis Herman, *Trauma and Recovery: The Aftermath of Violence—from Domestic Abuse to Political Terror* (New York: Basic Books, 2015), 173–74.
10. World Health Organization, *The International Classification of Diseases*, 11th ed., 2019, http://id.who.int/icd/entity/585833559.
11. Herman, *Trauma and Recovery*, 172.
12. See, for example, Marylène Cloitre et al., "Distinguishing PTSD, Complex PTSD, and Borderline Personality Disorder: A Latent Class Analysis," *European Journal of Psychotraumatology* 5 (2014): 1–10, doi: 10.3402/cjpt.v5.25097; Julian D. Ford and Christine A. Courtois, "Complex PTSD, Affect Dysregulation, and Borderline Personality Disorder," *Borderline Personality Disorder and Emotion Dysregulation* 1, no. 1 (2014): 1–17, doi: 10.1186/2051-6673-1-9.
13. Portions of the following section on the history and concepts of attachment theory are significantly reworked from a previously published work: Alexander Kriss, "An Abyss of Uncertainty: The Developmental Lines of Internal Working Models and Reflective Functioning," *Attachment and Complex Systems* 2, no. 1 (2015): 65–86.
14. John Bowlby, *Attachment and Loss*, vol. 1, *Attachment* (New York: Basic Books, 1969). See also his two sequel volumes: Bowlby, *Attachment and Loss*, vol. 2, *Separation* (New York: Basic Books, 1973); Bowlby, *Attachment and Loss*, vol. 3, *Loss* (New York: Basic Books, 1980).
15. Konrad Lorenz, "Der Kumpan in der Umwelt des Vogels / Der Artgenosse als auslösendes Moment sozialer Verhaltensweisen," *Journal für Ornithologie* 83 (1935): 137–215, 289–413.
16. Inge Bretherton, "Attachment Theory: Retrospect and Prospect," *Monographs of the Society for Research in Child Development* 50, nos. 1–2 (1985): 3–35.
17. Mary D. S. Ainsworth et al., *Patterns of Attachment: A Psychological Study of the Strange Situation* (Hillsdale, NJ: Earlbaum, 1978).

18. Peter Fonagy et al., "Measuring the Ghost in the Nursery: An Empirical Study of the Relation Between Parents' Mental Representations of Childhood Experiences and Their Infants' Security of Attachment," *Journal of the American Psychoanalytic Association* 41, no. 4 (1993): 957–89, doi: 10.1177/000306519304100403; Peter Fonagy et al., "Maternal Representations of Attachment During Pregnancy Predict the Organization of Infant-Mother Attachment at One Year of Age," *Child Development* 62 (1991): 891–905; Peter Fonagy et al., "The Capacity for Understanding Mental States: The Reflective Self in Parent and Child and Its Significance for Security of Attachment," *Infant Mental Health Journal* 12, no. 3 (1991): 201–18.

19. Mary Main and Judith Solomon, "Procedures for Identifying Infants as Disorganized/Disoriented During the Ainsworth Strange Situation," *Attachment in the Preschool Years: Theory, Research, and Intervention* (Chicago: University of Chicago Press, 1990), 121–60.

20. Karlen Lyons-Ruth et al., "Disorganized Infant Attachment Classification and Maternal Psychosocial Problems as Predictors of Hostile-Aggressive Behavior in the Preschool Classroom," *Child Development* 64 (1993): 572–85, doi: 10.1111/j.1467-8624.1993.tb02929.x.

21. Marinus H. van IJzendoorn et al., "Disorganized Attachment in Early Childhood: Meta-Analysis of Precursors, Concomitants, and Sequelae," *Development and Psychopathology* 11 (1999): 225–49.

22. For a review, see Vivien Prior and Danya Glaser, *Understanding Attachment and Attachment Disorders: Theory, Evidence and Practice* (Philadelphia: Jessica Kingsley Publishers, 2006).

23. Peter Fonagy et al., "Attachment, the Reflective Self, and Borderline States: The Predictive Specificity of the Adult Attachment Interview and Pathological Emotional Development," in *Attachment Theory: Social, Developmental and Clinical Perspectives*, ed. Susan Goldberg et al. (New York: Analytic Press, 1995), 233–78; Mary Main et al., "Studying Differences in Language Usage in Recounting Attachment History: An Introduction to the AAI," in *Clinical Applications of the Adult Attachment Interview*, ed. Howard Steele and Miriam Steele (New York: The Guilford Press, 2008), 31–68.

24. Van IJzendoorn et al., "Disorganized Attachment in Early Childhood."

25. Peter Fonagy, "Thinking About Thinking: Some Clinical and Theoretical Considerations in the Treatment of a Borderline Patient," *International Journal of Psychoanalysis* 72 (1991): 639–56; Peter Fonagy, "Playing with Reality: The Development of Psychic Reality and Its Malfunction in Borderline Personalities," *International Journal of Psychoanalysis* 76 (1995): 39–44.

26. Peter Fonagy, "Attachment and Borderline Personality Disorder," *Journal of the American Psychoanalytic Association* 48, no. 4 (2000): 1129–46, doi: 10.1177/00030651000480040701; Peter Fonagy et al., "The Developmental Roots of Borderline Personality Disorder in Early Attachment Relationships: A Theory and Some Evidence," *Psychoanalytic Inquiry* 23,

no. 3 (2003): 412–59; Peter Fonagy and Anthony Bateman, "The Development of Borderline Personality Disorder: A Mentalizing Model," *Journal of Personality Disorders* 22, no. 1 (2008): 4–12, doi: 10.1521/pedi .2008.22.1.4.

27. For a concise overview, see Michael Daubney and Anthony Bateman, "Mentalization-Based Therapy (MBT): An Overview," *Australasian Psychiatry* 23, no. 2 (2015), https://journals.sagepub.com/doi/full/10.1177 /1039856214566830.

28. Lois W. Choi-Kain and Brandon T. Unruh, "Mentalization-Based Treatment: A Common-Sense Approach to Borderline Personality Disorder," *Psychiatric Times* 33, no. 3 (2016), https://www.psychiatrictimes.com /view/mentalization-based-treatment-common-sense-approach-borderline -personality-disorder.

29. Anthony Bateman and Peter Fonagy, "Randomized Controlled Trial of Outpatient Mentalization-Based Treatment versus Structured Clinical Management for Borderline Personality Disorder," *American Journal of Psychiatry* 166 (2009): 1355–64; Trudie I. Rossouw and Peter Fonagy, "Mentalization-Based Treatment for Self-Harm in Adolescents: A Randomized Controlled Trial," *Journal of the American Academy of Child & Adolescent Psychiatry* 51, no. 12 (2012): 1304–13; Dave Carlyle et al., "A Randomized-Controlled Trial of Mentalization-Based Treatment Compared with Structured Case Management for Borderline Personality Disorder in a Mainstream Public Health Service," *Frontiers in Psychiatry* (November 12, 2020), https://www.frontiersin.org/articles/10.3389/fpsyt.2020.561916/full.

30. Stephan Doering et al., "Transference-Focused Psychotherapy v. Treatment by Community Psychotherapists for Borderline Personality Disorder: Randomised Controlled Trial," *British Journal of Psychiatry* 196 (2010): 389–95.

31. Anthony Bateman and Peter Fonagy, "Eight-Year Follow-Up of Patients Treated for Borderline Personality Disorder: Mentalization-Based Treatment versus Treatment as Usual," *American Journal of Psychiatry* 165 (2008): 631–38.

32. Herman, *Trauma and Recovery*, 281.

33. *DSM-5*, 761–63.

34. Thomas A. Widiger and Allen J. Frances, "Toward a Dimensional Model for the Personality Disorders," in *Personality Disorders and the Five-Factor Model of Personality*, ed. P. T. Costa and T. A. Widiger (Washington, DC: American Psychological Association, 2002): 23–44, doi: 10.1037/10423-003.

35. Carla Sharp and Joshua D. Miller, "Ten-Year Retrospective on the DSM-5 Alternative Model of Personality Disorder: Seeing the Forest for the Trees," *Personality Disorders: Theory, Research, and Treatment* 13, no. 4 (2022): 301–4, doi: 10.1037/per0000595.

36. *DSM-5*, 766–67.

37. *Psychodynamic Diagnostic Manual*, 2nd ed. (*PDM-2*), ed. Vittorio Lingiardi and Nancy McWilliams (New York: The Guilford Press, 2017), 15–29.

38. Clare Shaw and Gillian Proctor, "Women at the Margins: A Critique of the Diagnosis of Borderline Personality Disorder," *Feminism and Psychology* 15, no. 4 (November 2005): 487, doi: 10.1177/0959-353505057620.

39. More than one of my patients have cited the website "Out of the FOG" (https://outofthefog.website) as an especially helpful resource.

40. Abby Weems, Twitter, December 21, 2017, https://twitter.com/potty mouthworld/status/943999966304911360.

13: BORDERLINE

1. Jeremy D. Safran, Christopher Muran, and Bella Proskurov, "Alliance, Negotiation, and Rupture Resolution," in *Handbook of Evidence-Based Psychodynamic Psychotherapy: Bridging the Gap Between Science and Practice*, ed. Raymond A. Levy and J. Stuart Ablon (Totowa, NJ: Humana Press, 2009), 201–25.

INDEX